Praise for Juli
Skinny School and *Wife School:*

"What a great book!! I just love-love-love *Skinny School*!! I hate it's over. I want to read it again. Can't wait to share this treasure—truly a treasure—with all I can. I can't express enough how you have changed my life with these principles…You will touch women all over the world!" *Jeanne N.*

"*Skinny School* has literally changed my life. I feel amazing, and my light shines bright, meaning my inner joy and my love for people…I can only say that [*Skinny School*] is Truth. This book is so freeing." *Jan C.*

"Just finished reading your book. Love-love-love it! I especially love the way that it's written in fictional form. Awesome idea!" *Kerri G.*

"I just finished your book and I LOVED it. I am recommending it to all of my friends." Meredith G.

"I plan to encourage all of the women I know to read this book." *Rebecca P.*

"I keep ordering more copies. You won't know until heaven how many lives may be changed through you." *Kim M.*

"I am a hundred pages into your book. I can't put it down!" *Frieda K.*

"WIVES…do not miss!! Many of my friends are raving over Julie Gordon's book(s)." *Chyrll V.*

"You cannot imagine how much of a 'God-breath' this book is to me." *Amy M.*

"I especially like the format you've used employing fictional characters. It is much more enjoyable to read than a dry how-to book and hard to put down. I've already recommended it…" *Dena M.*

"I laughed out loud…I am buying this for our daughters…Wish I had had it years ago!!" *Judy F.*

"My daughter gave me a copy of your book for Christmas, and I read it in two days. I could not put it down. I bought several copies and sent them to people." *Sondra S.*

"I tried to make [the *Genie* book] last as long as possible because I did not want it to end! It was absolutely amazing…It will definitely be permanently placed in my night stand…Can't wait for your next book!" *Heather J.*

"When I first read your book, my world was rocked. I am now guiding a small group of women through your amazing book!" *Elizabeth L.*

"This book is written so creatively…Our pastor's wife came across your book…She was so impressed with your writing style and the way you changed her focus…The fruit yielded from such a short study was staggering." *Kelsey R.*

"A friend told me it was the best book she had read lately, so I read it over the summer. She was correct…" *Anne F.*

"I have read Julie's book twice now. It is AMAZING. I encourage all my girlfriends to read it and follow her blog. So insightful!" *Jennifer W.*

"I started reading Julie's book Saturday night and couldn't stop." *Chelsie G.*

"I really appreciated the style in which you wrote the book too. Since Jessica is transparent and real, it allowed me to see myself without defense—thank you! I loved your book! Buying one for all my friends!" *Francesca T.*

"I promise you, I have had girls [that I mentor] come back and say this book has changed their lives forever. I have ordered twelve more copies and am mailing them to my closest friends." *Debbie F.*

"Wish I would've read this eleven years ago. Best BOOK I have ever-ever read!" *Cherisse H.*

"Please allow me to say that when something touches you the way your book has me, it takes no effort at all to show appreciation! Your book has shed so much light on every aspect of my life...I could not stop reading!" *Tynesha K.*

"I wish I had Julie Gordon's [books] to follow at the beginning of my marriage: life-changing." *Cate C.*

"It helps me understand what is normal for women...I can't keep something this great to myself!!" *Emily K.*

"Your book truly has been life changing for me! I cannot thank you enough for writing this book." *Stephanie P.*

"Your book has helped me so much...Honestly, you have no idea. I have read AA books, codependency books, gone to AA meetings, church services, so on...but nothing got the pieces in the slots and the gears oiled and turning the way your book did. I feel alive for the first time in eight years...in EIGHT YEARS!" *Kristin M.*

"[My newest daughter-in-law] thanked me in all capital letters for giving [your book] to her! She began reading it and can't put it down!!! She said she loves it!" *Carol F.*

"Thank you for your book! It has truly changed me." *Stacy R.*

"I am so thankful for your book and online study. It has literally revolutionized me and is teaching me what my heart was longing for but just didn't know how or where to go to learn these godly truths." *Jill G.*

"Your guidance and knowledge are a godsend to me." *Kim B.*

"What a priceless gift I have through your book." *Erica V.*

"It has been an amazing gift, and it's unlike anything else I have read." *Jessica B.*

Skinny School: Where Women Learn the Secrets to Finally Get Thin Forever

Skinny School: Where Women Learn the Secrets to Finally Get Thin Forever

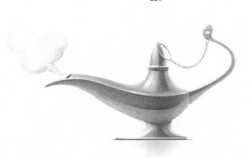

Julie N Gordon
MS, Marriage and Family Counseling

Cover design by Bhovidhya Pawan
Copyright © 2015 Julie N. Gordon
All rights reserved.

ISBN: 0692370722
ISBN 13: 9780692370728

Although every effort has been made to ensure that the contents of this book are accurate, it must not be treated as a substitute for qualified medical advice. The author cannot be held responsible for any loss or claim arising out of the use, or misuse, of any of the suggestions made or the failure to take medical advice. The purpose of this book is to educate. This information is in no way intended as a substitute for medical counseling.

Skinny School is Book Two in the
Genie School Series for Women

Book One:
Wife School: Where Women Learn the Secrets of Making Husbands Happy
(available at Amazon.com and other online booksellers)

Book Three in this series will be:
Happy School: Where Women Learn the Secrets of Thinking Correctly about
What is Missing and Disappointing in Their Lives

Currently being written (with coauthor David Gordon):
Husband School, Where Men Learn the Secret Codes that Unlock A Wife's Soul

Table of Contents

If you do not like the title Skinny School...

Yes, yes, I have been told that *skinny* is not a good word for the title. To some, it speaks of unhealthy body image issues—maybe even anorexia or bulimia. I am well aware of this severe problem in young women.

However, *skinny* is simply a word that today's woman likes. If a two-hundred-pound woman slims down to 175 pounds, her friends will say, "You look skinny." The word does not always mean the emaciated-runway-model look. *Skinny* is a fun word that women know and love.

Recently a woman who is five foot two told me she thought 150 pounds was a good weight for her. Another woman who is five foot nine said that 126 pounds was her best weight. I realized once again that *our personal goals vary a lot*. You set your own goal. Whatever is skinny for you is great with this program.

Being a Christian, I am well aware of the secular culture's obsession with outward beauty versus a lack of focus on inner beauty. Friend! Of course, inner beauty should be our focus, but that does not negate the need for *self-control and healthy eating*. Just know that this program is as much about eating healthy as it is about eating to get thin.

If you have struggled with your weight, then you know how much energy your problem takes away from your ability to focus outwardly. The *Skinny School* program will get *overeating* off your list—and then watch your energy to love and give to others soar!

Again, I am sorry if the word *skinny* offends you. Please overlook it and enjoy these principles that will enable you to get healthy and thin.

And, BTW, the model on the cover is a cartoon, not a real person. *Cartoons are often exaggerated to make a point.*

Preface

By flipping the switch in how to think, women in *Skinny School* are able to shed thirty, fifty, seventy, or more pounds. This is done by getting inside a woman's head with knowledge and logic so she can reason within herself. Once a woman gets it, she is forever free from her insanity eating. Freedom from overeating—and the subsequent attainment of thinness—is exhilarating!

From surveying the women I have counseled and mentored over the past twenty-five years, I've concluded that the top three issues with which Christian women repeatedly struggle are (1) their dissatisfaction in marriage, (2) their weight, and (3) the feeling of being shackled with a discouraged, unhappy heart. My first book, *Wife School: Where Women Learn the Secrets to Making Husbands Happy*, featured a bratty and abrasive protagonist, Jessica, who learned the secrets to making her marriage sing. In this second book of the Genie series, *Skinny School: Where Women Learn the Secrets of Finally Getting Thin Forever*, the single, savvy, but chubby protagonist, Jackie (who is Jessica's younger sister), learns the coveted secrets to finally being thin forever.

As a teen, a young adult, and once again in my forties, I struggled with excess weight. The agony a woman feels in dealing with being overweight is one of the most discouraging and heartbreaking trials that women experience. (If you disagree, then you have never severely struggled with your weight.) Having read over a thousand books on this topic, I feel it is only in the last few years that I finally learned the last piece of the skinny puzzle (ditching sugars and starches, Lesson Two). As you will discover, *weight loss is all about retraining the mind in thinking about and eating food so one can therefore make the right choices.*

In *Skinny School*, I write about the science of weight loss by quoting experts in the field (see Appendix D for a list of these health gurus). But my specific spin in *Skinny School* will be to help you get your mind in the right place, the mind of a Champion, the mind that wants—and is able to—trade temporary pleasure for a higher goal.

Now hear this glorious truth: you can learn these *Skinny School* lessons just like you learned math facts. If you can learn to type, you can learn these lessons. You will change how you think, and therefore you will be in charge of whether you eat those M&M's or even have that unneeded second helping of something healthy. This program will take effort, time, and energy to learn, but after all, this is something you really, truly want. Right?

In a way similar to how the authors of *Charlotte's Web*, *The Velveteen Rabbit,* and *The Lion, the Witch and the Wardrobe* used toys and animals to speak profound truths, I have used a Genie to convey wisdom in this story. He is not the goofy Genie of Disney or the silly Genie played by Shaq; this Genie is a wise and relentless counselor who instructs the protagonist how to finally get thin forever.

Please visit my website at www.JulieNGordon.com/SkinnySchool to find the Genie recipes and many other resources to help you.

I wish I had known these truths at fifteen years old; I would have spared myself much suffering. These strategies have enabled the women in my groups to retrain their brains so that there is a "flip" and a "click" where they now view food and eating differently and are subsequently able to get thin. This program works.

Are you ready to transform your life?

Dear Reader, please read these five remarks before beginning *Skinny School*.

1. *Skinny School* is written in a story format to make it enjoyable. However, it is meant to be used as a workbook. Please get your colored pens and highlighters out and mark up this book. It will be imperative that you read—and reread—and reread again—the remarks of the Genie until the new thinking becomes your own. The Genie's remarks in each lesson are listed in the table of contents, and they are announced in each lesson with a bold typeface so you can easily locate the Genie portion to reread.

2. The Genie asks Jackie to do assignments and keep them in her Ruby Journal. Any notebook will do, but the importance of doing and accumulating these assignments is the difference between failure and huge success.

3. You are going to fail on this program at first. It is everyone's path. But the secret is to *keep rereading the Genie's thinking and to work in your Ruby Journal.* Lesson Seven is on failure. Since you will fail, you must have a strategy for getting back on the bus quickly. Do not become discouraged if you fail. After you read Lesson Seven on failure, you will better understand. Perseverance is magical.

4. A twenty-three-week online course, *Skinny School Online* (currently free), will be offered periodically. Check JulieNGordon.com for dates

of upcoming sessions. These lessons will be e-mailed to your inbox weekly. (The women who have taken the free twenty-two-week on-line course *Wife School Online*, in addition to reading the book *Wife School*, quantumly increased their success in transforming their marriages.) In addition to accessing free classes on her website, you can sign up for Julie's blog and new book release announcements, enjoy many recipes, and discover a host of other valuable information.

5. This last suggestion may be the most important one. For best results, find three to five other women to meet with weekly to discuss this material. Research has repeatedly shown that a group hugely contributes to success when trying to change behavior. See Appendix F for a group reading guide.

Dedicated to Elizabeth

"Her presence lights the home; her approach is like a cheerful warmth; she passes by and we are content; she stays a while and we are happy."
From *Toilers of the Sea* by Victor Hugo

The Nine Secrets of Finally Getting Thin Forever

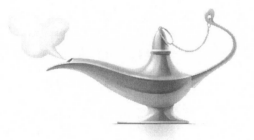

Lesson 1

Get in Touch with
Your Current Top Four Life Goals

Tuesday, August 12   *Weight: 175*   *Need to lose: 45 pounds*

My nervousness is apparent in every corner of my body. I glance in the rear-view mirror for one last check to see if I need to reapply lipstick or powder my incessantly shiny nose. My hair and makeup look adequate. Glancing down at my body, I figure I have camouflaged these excess forty-five pounds as well as I can, wearing these new black pants with the matching long tunic.

Opening the car door, I take a huge breath and gaze up at the impressive, cream stucco building with MICHAEL E. SIMPSON LAW embossed elegantly above the front doors. The building in its grandeur is even intimidating.

Beth Willibanks, who is my best friend, recently had her first baby, Alexis, and is now a stay-at-home mom. Her husband, Richard, is the bookkeeper/accountant at the Michael E. Simpson Law office and is best friends with the firm's young all-star attorney, Zach Boltz. I almost feel like I know Zach, as Beth has talked about him for months, along with the hilarious stories of his stuck-up girlfriend, Rachel. Repeatedly Beth has said she cannot believe that Zach would date such a snob, but we both agreed that men can be idiots when it comes to beautiful women. Anyhow, Beth told me yesterday that Richard said Zach's current legal assistant gave her two weeks' notice because she is moving back to Dallas to be near her family. Beth knows I have been looking for another legal assistant job for a few months. Although I like my current boss, Mr. Fortwright, he has had alcohol issues for years, and it is just a matter of time until his practice goes under. I have been keeping the Titanic of his law practice afloat for over four years. Actually, I do everything in Mr. Fortwright's practice except show up in court. And when it is time to show up in court on one of his cases, Mr. Fortwright has missed more appearances than I want to count. He does pay me extremely well, but his ship is getting ready to hit an iceberg, and I do not want to be stranded when it does. Beth said she and Richard think the job of being Zach Boltz's legal assistant will be a perfect fit for me. Hence my interview in ten minutes. I am shaky, I am so nervous.

Walking into the reception area, I am struck by the ageless beauty of the traditional successful law firm, the dark wood, gold trim, and leather sofas. This lobby is quite a contrast to the faded, plaid wingback chairs in Fortright's foyer. I immediately feel out of place.

Glancing into the gold-gilded mirror in the foyer, I notice my long blond hair and a decent-looking face staring back at me (I am grateful for my mother's wide-set eyes and her little turned-up nose). But below that is my chunky self. Here I am, in the youthful prime of life, the time when life is supposed to be light and happy, the time when one dates and marries her life partner, and I am instead cursed with this weight and insanity eating.

Wrestling my mind back from that digression, I turn to look at the girl behind the massive mahogany reception desk. Barely glancing my direction, she mumbles, "May I help you?"

Beth—having a proclivity for knowing all the latest drama in all of her social circles—had already warned me about Eva, the receptionist, who also happens to be the Attorney Michael E. Simpson's daughter. Beth said that Eva likes to play her boss's-daughter card, acting as if she has been endowed with high authority, when in truth she is merely the company gofer, answering the phone and opening mail. Renee—the current legal assistant who is moving and who is chubby like me—said that Eva's heel height may be high, but her IQ is low. A mean remark, I admit, but I have noticed that we chubby girls like to make fun of skinny twig girls. Obviously, it is just an ugly and wrong technique to deal with our jealousies.

Judging from this side of the desk, Eva appears to be around a hundred pounds. Her smoky eye makeup is subtle and discreetly applied, and her long, brown, bouncy hair has been perfectly highlighted. She has on a tight-fitting, bright yellow knit shirt with a soft, dainty necklace. Her perfume is light, flowery, and friendly, quite the contrast to her condescending and suspicious vibes. Obviously, she is the royal gatekeeper.

"I am Jackie Holbrook, and I have an appointment at eleven with Zach Boltz," I say in my most perky voice, trying to ignore her unfriendliness.

"Oh, so you are interviewing for Zach's assistant, are you?" Her eyes travel up and down my body before they come back to meet my eyes.

Suddenly, I wish I was not applying for this stupid job, even though I am extremely qualified. I wish I was back at my old comfortable job at Fortwright's, where there are not any snotty stick receptionists to make me feel frumpy and second class.

"Follow me," she says, as if she is the prison warden and I am a new inmate. She rises from her seat and begins her descent down the hall. She leads with her legs, which jut out from under a skirt that is four inches above her bony knees. Her yellow four-inch wedges are further making me wish I had told Beth that I did not want to interview here. The picture of Eva and me must be similar to a toy poodle with ribbons, fresh from the manicurist, leading a pregnant St. Bernard.

Breathing deeply, I follow her, wishing I was anywhere but here. The toothpick boss's daughter points toward the open door and I enter, not knowing what else to do, like an ox being led to slaughter. What an idiot I am to think that a highbrow law firm like this would want a toad like me. Why did I let Beth talk me into this? I belong in a law office with faded, plaid wingback chairs.

Entering the office, I see Zach Boltz, who is a cross between the deceased John F. Kennedy, Jr., and Chris Pine. My first impression of Zach reminds me of a man on a sailboat in Martha's Vineyard, dressed in Ralph Lauren, checking his net worth periodically on his phone. Although Beth had told me about Zach's driving work ethic and his no-nonsense personality, she failed to warn me about his Ivy League good looks. Beth has talked often of Rachel, Zach's polished and cultivated girlfriend, as she and Richard have double dated with Zach and Rachel a couple of times. But Beth does not like Rachel, as she feels as though Rachel acts as if she is in a superior class of females. Beth says Rachel carries Kate Spade purses, wears Burberry coats, and spends her time on some part-time public relations job, playing tennis and getting facials with the other hours. Must be nice.

Zach is friendly enough but all business. "This is quite a list of jobs that you perform for Fortwright," he comments, while reading my résumé. "Most legal assistants do not do all these tasks."

I know I could reveal Fortwright's problem and consequently why I was forced to learn so much law, but it is not necessary, and I suddenly feel a strange loyalty to Fortwright.

"Mr. Fortwright likes me to take care of almost everything in the office," I say. Zach studies me as I answer, waiting for more information, but it does not come. And he does not pry. He nods as if no further explanation is needed.

Instantly, I begin to relax in front of this nonjudgmental, composed guy. I forget about the twig receptionist, and I am able to calm down in the presence of this man who is judging me on what I would bring to the job, not on how I would look on a runway. He tells me about what he needs; I tell him how I can accomplish his work.

Forty short minutes later, Zach offers me the job (having Richard and Beth's referral did not hurt things), and we agree to start the day after Labor Day so that I can give a proper two weeks' notice to Mr. Fortwright. I already feel sad for Mr. Fortwright. With me resigning, I hope he will enter recovery.

"Follow me," Zach says. "We need to go through the formality of introducing you to Attorney Simpson."

Attorney Simpson's image, as I see him on his TV ads all the time, pops into my mind. He looks like the quintessential successful attorney, sporting a thick head of gray hair, a thousand-dollar suit, and a trim body that hints at a personal trainer who counts while he does push-ups.

Following Zach down the hall, we enter a monstrous, palatial-like room on the other side of the foyer where Attorney Simpson sits at his desk, or more accurately, on his throne. Attorney Simpson is polite but obviously busy, and the formality of meeting the head honcho is quickly over. Zach accompanies me back to the foyer, where Little Miss Lemon Wedges is sorting the mail.

"Eva, you already met my new assistant, Jackie, didn't you?" Zach asks.

Immediately, a sly smile crosses her face. "We met," she says. "Jackie, I have invited all the young people in the office over to my apartment to swim and cook out around noon on Saturday. We would love for you to join us."

Swim? As in swimsuit? *Swimsuit* is the most despicable word in the English language to a fattie. I can see it now: Little Miss Lemon Wedges in her polka-dot bikini and me, Miss Bullfrog, in my one-piece black swimsuit with the skirt that tries to hide my cannon thighs. Uh, no thanks.

"I have plans, but thank you anyhow," I say, lying in my sweetest voice.

"Aw, that is too bad," she says in a pouty voice. Then Eva giggles and turns to Zach. "Zach, maybe you will bring some free Chick-Fil-A for all of us to eat."

I do not get what is so funny about bringing Chick-Fil-A.

"You will have to ask Rachel," he says, expressionless, before retreating to his office to get back to work.

Renee, the current legal assistant who is leaving, walks up at that moment and, hearing the comment, giggles with Eva at the remark. This must be some inside joke, and I certainly do not get it. Renee begins to explain, "Zach is dating Rachel, and her father owns a couple Chick-Fil-As in Nashville. We like to harass Zach for free food." Renee and Eva both giggle again.

A creepy feeling begins to rise in my stomach. Beth and I have discussed Rachel many times, and she never mentioned that Rachel's father owned Chick-Fil-As. I knew a girl in high school named Rachel whose dad owned Chick-Fil-As, but of course, that was Memphis and this is Nashville. And of course, that was ten years ago, and Rachel is such a common name, so I know it is a different Rachel. It is ridiculous to ask, but just for fun, just for my peace of mind, I will ask.

"What is Rachel's last name?"

Silly of me to ask because, of course, it is Smith...or O'Henry...or Timberlake. No way it is Hanover.

"Hanover," Eva says.

The drop in the stomach is like the drop you feel when you go over the top on a roller coaster. A wave of desperation sweeps over me. *Rachel Hanover? My new boss is dating Rachel Hanover?*

Thoughts of high school flood my brain. I was somewhat *socially* invisible in high school, although I was a very good student. There were over eight hundred students in my graduating class, of which Rachel was one of the popular ones. I was one of the, eh, chubby ones. I got mononucleosis in my junior year and used that illness as an excuse to miss many days over the next two years. Really, I skipped school all the time, mainly because I was miserable watching the cute guys flirt with the cute girls. I agonized when they whispered about their weekend plans, from which, of course, I was excluded. I still cannot believe my mother let me skip school like I did. But even with all the absences, my teachers felt sorry for my "illness" and let me out of doing many of the assignments. Somehow, I kept making As.

During the fall of my senior year, I lost around thirty pounds, and one weekend, I had thirteen guys ask me out. Thirteen offers for one weekend! One of the invitations was to a Christmas dance with a popular (but dorky) football player. He was in the in crowd so at the dance, we all sat around a huge round table with our Cokes and Sprites (which I think also had other substances in most of them). Rachel was at that table with all of her gang, and I do not think I spoke to a single one of them the entire night. *I* was the new girl—shouldn't they be friendly first?

In high school, Rachel was surrounded by her popular drill team buddies; I was surrounded by my spiral notebooks, filled with unmet dreams.

Many classmates thought Rachel was a natural beauty in a classic sense. Actually, I thought she was a little bug-eyed, but I am sure jealousy played a role in that evaluation. To me, it seemed as though Rachel's goal in life was to attain maximum social status, not having any margins for kids who were in the second or third tier of popularity.

Frequently, Rachel and I used to pass each other in the halls at school. One day I saw her coming down the student-crammed hall, saying hi to this girl, and then giggling at another guy's remark. When she got to me, I was ready to robustly smile and say the friendliest hello I knew how to say.

But when she reached me in the hall, she averted her eyes, like suddenly she had to think about something important, like maybe she forgot her physics homework. That was the last time I tried to connect with popular Rachel.

Of course, I understood why Rachel could not see me. She truly was in a different social stratum, after all. She was one of the captains of the drill team; I was in the French club. She dated one of the popular football players; I did not date much period. We were both in honors English, though, and I remember one class in which the teacher asked the class to say what they would invent, if they could invent anything, no limitations whatsoever. After a few other classmates gave their suggestions, I raised my hand and said that I would invent a pill that was worth eight hours of sleep. That is, I continued to explain, you would have all the physical, mental, and emotional benefits even though you did not have to sleep, thus regaining eight more hours in each day. The teacher loved the idea, and many of my classmates said they thought that was the best idea yet. I happened to hear someone behind me whisper, "Then there would be more time to eat banana splits." I turned to see who said it. It was not Rachel; it was her giggling cohort friend, but there was Rachel, snickering and enjoying the humor. Rachel was smart like that; she did not say the mean stuff, but she certainly enjoyed it.

At the end of my senior year, I was tied for valedictorian (yes, even with missing so much school); Rachel was tied for Most Beautiful. Often when I entered the senior lounge, Rachel would be on a sofa with her legs pulled up to her chest and her arms around her knees, sort of to show the world how little space she occupied when bunched all together.

Another one of her favorite positions was sitting on the sofa with her shoes off and her legs curled up under her, as again, putting herself in a tiny box. I often thought what a cow I would look like in either of those positions.

The one time that Rachel approached me in all of high school was near the end of our senior year. "Do you want to buy some tickets to a private dance after graduation?" she asked.

Why, I was immediately flattered. *Rachel Hanover is asking me to a private after-graduation party!* Maybe I had arrived socially after all. Maybe I was finally being included. I even wondered if she and I might hang out that last summer a little, before we all separated for college.

But later, I found out her high school sorority was sponsoring the dance, and she was chairman of the event, obviously just trying to ratchet up ticket sales. There was absolutely nothing in that request about acceptance or arrival or friendship or any other dunce thought that I might have had—only her gain by making her event successful with numbers, even if that meant inviting nobody me.

The horror of the whole current situation is now unraveling before my eyes. I am going to work for Rachel Hanover's boyfriend. Zach walks back out of his office and hands Eva some packages to mail.

"Do you know Rachel?" Eva asks me in front of Zach.

"Uh, maybe," I say. "I went to high school in Memphis with a girl named Rachel Hanover." Please, please, please, let this be a different Rachel Hanover.

"Yes, the Hanovers are from Memphis," Zach says matter-of-factly. "They moved here ten years ago. Small world." Zach expeditiously returns to his office again.

Walking to my car, I feel a knot in my stomach that feels like I just found out my puppy died. Rachel Hanover is alive and in Nashville to haunt me again.

Pulling out of the parking lot, all my prior happiness at getting this new job dissipates as anxiety sets in. I think of all the skinny Rachels in life who are born into family and money and who date guys like Zach Boltz but cannot seem to see me. Yeah, I am smart, maybe even kind of pretty on a good day, and definitely hard working. But dang it, being fat puts me in another class of women! I hate-hate-hate being fat!

Just like a million times before, I decide that tomorrow I will begin my journey to join the Skinny Club of America, and this time, tomorrow will be different. Tomorrow, I will only eat lettuce and broccoli and maybe occasionally some broiled chicken. Tomorrow, I will starve myself, no matter what, until I am a beanpole. Tomorrow I will sign up for boot camp at 5:00 a.m. five times a week! These pronouncements and declarations of tomorrow's diet and exercise program make me feel temporarily somewhat better.

But anyhow, that is tomorrow's plan. Therefore today, I may as well enjoy myself one last time. I speed to my favorite fast-food drive-through restaurant and get the works: double cheeseburger, large fries, and a chocolate shake. Eating in my car, I am finished by the time I get to my apartment. The fullness from such a binge makes me temporarily forget about Eva's bony knees and Rachel's past condescension. The familiar sense of hopelessness and discouragement entangles me again as it predictably does after I fall prey to a binge.

Arriving at my apartment, I notice there is a package in the doorway. I pick it up and carry it into my apartment. That is strange; there is no return address on the box.

Opening the package, I discover a mahogany box. I then proceed to open this box, and inside lies an old brass lamp with a handle and a spout. It looks like it belonged to Aladdin. Is this some kind of joke? Who would send me this junk?[1]

Picking up the Aladdin-like lamp, I notice there is a cork in the spout. Maybe the gift-giver left a note inside the lantern. I remove the cork from the spout, and a pillar of smoke arises. Immediately, I am petrified. Dropping the lamp on the sofa, I run into the hall to escape what I fear is going to be an explosion. There is no explosion, so I peek back around the corner.

Standing in my den is a dark, middle-aged Middle Eastern man. He is around six feet tall and looks like he has worked out every day of his life. His tanned skin looks a little dry, like men who are sailors or who have played tennis without sunscreen all their lives. His eyebrows are a little on the bushy side, but they make his face interesting. His most surprising feature is his gaze—soft and filled with kindness, free of any malice. Gold silk pants are topped with a white vest embroidered with gold thread, and a large turban populated with sparkly gems sits on his head.

Seeing me, he motions for me to come to him. **"Do not be afraid, Young Jackie. I am your Genie and am now here to grant you one wish."**

---

1 If you have read *Wife School, Where Women Learn the Secrets of Making Husbands Happy,* you will remember that Jackie's sister, Jessica, has anonymously sent her the Genie.

Petrified, I wonder how this criminal got in. The doors are locked, and the alarm is on. Is this a dream? I slap my thigh, but I do not wake up.

"It is true," he continues. "I am your Genie, and I am here to grant you a wish, Young Jackie. What do you wish?"

How does he know my name? Who is this? My heart rate must be two hundred, but his calm eyes tell me I am safe. Beginning to calm down, I slowly move toward him.

"Go ahead. Tell me your one wish, Young Jackie."

After ten more minutes of this repetitive dialogue where I question him, touch him, and slap myself again to wake myself up, I realize that if this is a dream, I will eventually wake up, so I might as well go along with his instructions. Thoughts of beanpole Eva and her tiny hips that are barely wider than a single piece of spaghetti explode into my brain. Coming up with the right wish is an easy choice.

"Genie, my one wish is this: I want to be skinny!"

I close my eyes, waiting to feel the electric tingle of shrinking from a size eighteen to a size four. I wait. I wait a little more.

Opening my eyes, I think that maybe one does not feel the shrinking when a Genie does an abracadabra on you. I gaze down to see my new tiny body. But my pig-like gut is still there. What is up with that? What kind of Genie is this?

"Are you ready to begin your lessons in *Skinny School*?" the Genie asks.

"Uh, waaiiiit a minute," I say. "What lessons? I don't want any lessons. I want to be skinny. Right now."

"Your wish is to be skinny," he says. "If I just zap you, then you would still have the same thoughts and beliefs, and in no time, you would be back at your current weight because you would return to your present habits. I am not going to do a short-term fix. I am going to train your mind in *how to think about food and eating*, and therefore, you will be thin the rest of your life."

How lame is this? I ask for skinniness, and he is enrolling me in some dumb school?

"The only thing you need in order to change your weight forever is to change how you *think about food*," he says. "Currently, when you look at a piece of chocolate cake, you immediately have a thought about the cake. Your thought is something like, 'Oh, that would taste delicious. I want that right now.'"

This guy is a regular genius. Wow, he knows I want chocolate cake when I see it. A four-year-old could have told me that.

"A woman who has been through my *Skinny School* course will have a different thought when she looks at the cake. This woman will see the chocolate cake as *adversely* affecting her hormones, which drives her body's tendency to store fat. She will see the cake *negatively* nourishing her body for optimum health at a cellular level. My *Skinny School* graduate will recognize the emotional freedom and stability she now experiences since she is no longer addicted to sugar. And lastly, my student understands that this act of immediate gratification—eating the chocolate cake—actually keeps her from reaching her true goals: health and thinness. These are only a few of the new thoughts you will learn as you study the secrets in *Skinny School*, where you will acquire freedom from overeating. These secrets will virtually give you back your life, the life that food and being overweight have stolen from you over the past years."

Who can believe how much time, energy, and despair I have wasted over the last thirteen years because of my fight with food and weight? But still, I bet his dumb secrets are as empty as all the other ones I have tried.

"In *Skinny School*, we will study the secrets women need to know to permanently pull themselves out of the overweight ditch forever."

Oh, dear. He thinks his little dopey secrets are going to fix my intricate, complicated, extremely convoluted and sophisticated relationship with food. This Genie has escaped from an asylum. And I should be locked up in one for listening to him.

"The lessons in *Skinny School* are not complicated, and they will enable you to quit making your weight the center of your universe. My method is permanent freedom from food forever without years of therapy. And you will enjoy food more than you ever have before."

Surely he is not boiling this complex situation with my obsession with food into some easy one-two-three answers. Yeah, sure, a few secrets and I will be free from this torture. I should know better than to take advice from someone who looks like he just left a Halloween party.

"To get started, you will need a journal to collect the thoughts and principles of all of your new lessons," he says as he whisks his hand into the air and a beautiful, gem-covered ruby journal appears. The journal is opulent and looks more like a journal for Princess Kate than for middle-class me. "The lists in this Ruby Journal will become your coach, your counselor, and your encourager, who will be available to you twenty-four-seven. By daily reading your Ruby Journal, you will *retrain your mind to think differently* about food and eating."

Why have these secrets not been on *The Biggest Loser* if they are so amazing? I never read this stuff in *People* magazine.

"We will now discuss the first aspect of today's lesson," he says, "which is: *do you truly care about being thin?*"

Do I truly care about being thin?! I am a woman. I am breathing. I live in America. That answers that question right there.

"Please entitle page one in your Ruby Journal 'My Top Four Life Goals,'" he says as he hands me the journal. "Then, in no particular order, I want you to brainstorm all the possible life goals you have *right now*. After that, I want you to star your top four goals."

Eh, I am a little confused. I did not ask for a life coach; I asked to be skinny. Maybe my Genie is a little hard of hearing.

"I am trying to understand why we are listing life goals when all I want is to be a waif," I say, trying to get out of his nonsense assignment.

"Getting in touch with your current Top Four Life Goals is a very important first step in Skinny School. You realize that for someone to become a world-class pianist, one would *not* expect them to also strive at the same time to be a multiple-times *New York Times* bestselling author as well as an excellent trial attorney."

What in the world does this have to do with size four jeans?

"Would it not be equally ludicrous if a woman wanted to simultaneously run a huge corporation, raise a family of six children, and train for the

Olympics? We would all immediately see the insanity of trying to accomplish all of those goals at the same time. Wisdom would tell her to pick what is *most* important to her and focus on that. Humans are finite creatures and can only accomplish so much. They have to narrow their focus if they want to be productive and successful at their endeavors."

Ooooh…kayyyy…But how does this relate to me and my goal of having hips like Eva? I still do not get the connection.

"People are too scattered in their goals, and by *not* focusing on doing a *few* things well, they do *nothing* well. Pick four goals—or five or six at the *very* most—and then let other goals go for now. *Taking massive action daily on a few select goals is the secret to accomplishing them.*"

I am not sure he is right on this. I can do more than four measly goals. Why, right now, I am studying for the LSAT, working full-time, attempting to have a vast social life (ha, what a joke), learning to grow flowers in pots on my patio, helping disadvantaged kids with their homework one night a week (well, I will start again when the school year starts), taking painting lessons, and learning French online. Having multiple interests makes me an interesting person, doesn't it? This Genie guy is saying that I am scattered and therefore not doing anything very well. That is not right, is it?

Immediately I think of my flowers dying on my patio, the canvas waiting with the beginnings of painting, and my online French lessons standing by for weeks.

"Young Jackie, as I said, it is time to get focused. Let us figure out the current Top Four Life Goals you have as you see them right now, and we will let other goals go for now. Again, write down every possible goal you can think of, and then we will prioritize the top four."

Still thinking this is a dumb dream, I decide I will go along with it. I write down fifteen items that I might have as goals right now. Included in the list are taking a course in novel writing and visiting my Memphis family more.

"Good job," he says. "Now, look down that list and pick the four most important goals you want to work on right now."

He is sort of pushy.

"I want to make my Creator happy," I say, thinking of who I am in my faith at my deepest core. That goal has several dimensions to it, such as prayer and studying the Creator's Word, but I will think about all of that later.

"Star that goal," the Genie says.

I star it.

"I want to marry the man of my dreams and have a lovely family someday," I say, but a sinking feeling wells up in me when I think of my current boyfriend, Robert, and how he does not fit the description of "man of my dreams." I will have to deal with that unpleasant thought later.

"Star that goal, too," he again says, interrupting my discouraging thoughts about Robert.

"I want to find work that I truly love and that benefits others," I say, shifting my thoughts to my recent efforts to study for the LSAT. (Actually, what I would *really* like is to be a novelist, but that is out of the question because I would never be able to support myself.)

"Excellent," he continues. "Star that goal too. What else?"

The goal that has *not* been said but that is definitely in the top four spews out: "I want to be thin and healthy for the rest of my life!"

The Genie's sly smile tells me he is not surprised.

"What I wanted you to see in that exercise," the Genie says, "is that you *seriously, truly care* about this goal of being thin and healthy. You need to realize how hugely important this goal is to you. It is not some little add-on thing. Being thin and healthy for the rest of your life is right up there with your relationship with the Creator, finding the right life partner, and discovering your life work. In your opinion, this goal *is central and imperative to your sense of well-being* as well as what you want during your short time here on earth."

Uh, I already knew that, Your Highness.

"This clarity often helps women see that their top goals do not include decorating their houses, running the PTA, or smocking the cutest baby clothes. These might be legitimate activities, but they are not likely in their current Top Four Life Goals. Women need to hear themselves admit out loud how much *they truly care* about permanently solving their weight struggles.

And then *women need to streamline and narrow their goals to only a few*, or else they will be scattered and get nothing accomplished."

Every time I see a thin woman, I wince with depasse. Maybe that is jealousy or discontent or who-knows-what, but I long to be thin. I loathe being a frump.

"What is so magnificent about hearing yourself say that being thin and healthy is in your current Top Four Life Goals is that it *frees you* to heavily invest for a season to study and learn the subject, applying massive amounts of effort to master the material, and thus *reprograming your mind* about food and eating. You will not have to focus and give this much attention to the subject forever, but for now, at this stage, this Herculean effort will be needed to override your current wrong thinking pattern. *I also want you to consider laying aside some of your other goals at this season*, so you can focus on relearning how to think about food and eating."

Something feels unsettling and selfish in spending this much effort on something that is all about me. "It seems a little trivial to ask to be skinny with all the problems in the world," I say, embarrassed. Now I think I should have said "solving world hunger" when I listed my top life goals. Again, I am such a loser.

Sensing my guilt, the Genie says, "If you have a continual struggle in an area, it is not wrong or shallow to want to find answers to solve that problem. If you are overweight, you are not healthy, and you cannot serve the Creator if you are in the grave. It is a lie that it is shallow to be concerned with health and achieving an appropriate weight. I want you to be free from that wrong thinking, so you can invest the needed time and energy to relearn the subject of eating and food. The truth is that after you have conquered this problem, you will have much more energy to help solve other people's problems and serious social dilemmas."

That helps. My guilt about applying so much energy to losing weight is one excuse I have used to ignore this problem.

"The second part of Lesson One today is, *are you willing to do the work to learn this new way of thinking?* As you know, in most endeavors, you humans expect to work and greatly persevere to accomplish your top important life goals," he says. "For example, to accomplish the goal of becoming a doctor, we all understand that much studying is required, and by necessity, recurring late nights of playing pool with the gang must be eliminated. How ludicrous for a medical student to say that she wants to be a doctor without giving up many pleasurable activities in favor of large amounts of study and diligent effort."

That is a stupid example. Of course, medical students must study and give up hanging out. And is that not overkill to compare losing weight to going to medical school?

"People who want to compete at the Olympics train for hours a day and do not bemoan the fact that they do not get to hang out at the mall or stay up late watching old movies. They have a goal, and they realize that the sacrifice of other pleasurable activities is needed to reach goals," he continues.

Again, his illustration is ridiculous. "Genie, this is losing weight, not the Olympics," I say, hoping he doesn't read any disrespect into my bold objection. "It feels a little foolish to put my personal weight loss up there in the categories like becoming a doctor or entering the Olympics."

"But did you not hear yourself?" he asks. "Being thin and healthy *is what is important to you.* Your desire to lose weight is no different from those people's top goals. What is different is they want something badly, and they know that to achieve it, *they must do the work.*"

I do not know what moronic work he is talking about. But he is right that I want to be skinny. However, I have always thought my weight problem was genetic…or that it was because I have some Italian blood and I am intensely passionate…or because, well, because of something that is *not* my fault.

"Of course, you have an obstacle before you, which is relearning how to think about food and eating. But let me remind you that life is full of obstacles. I will not allow you to indulge in self-pity. Some people, Young Jackie, are blinded by accidents. They are then required to learn Braille and live without sight the rest of their lives. Do you know that many people do this cheerfully, without self-pity or anger?" he says.

Oh, no. Surely he is not comparing the fact that I stuff my face to someone coping with being blind, is he?

"Another example of people conquering obstacles in their lives is how some people lose their legs in accidents and still decide to participate with stellar attitudes in activities, such as wheelchair basketball," he says.

Why is he comparing such heroic examples to my insanity with overeating?

"And do not forget the example of someone from poverty," he says, "who, through tenacious grit, plods, plows, fights, and does whatever it takes to overcome her negative circumstances so she can get her education."

I feel like a jerk, an A1 jerk, having a self-centered eating problem when these heroic individuals conquer huge obstacles with their indomitable spirits. What in the world do I have in common with all these examples of people with gigantic handicaps?

"In life, all humans have difficult issues to overcome," he says. "And if others can overcome their very difficult situations by using *elite Champion thinking, enormous effort, repeated sacrifice, and unwavering perseverance,* than you too can learn these secrets and apply them for overcoming your hardship with your excess weight."

This is a little weird. I am expecting a twelve-hundred-calorie diet with a workout program. He is saying the way to overcome my weight issue is through training my brain to think like an elite Champion. Surely I am going to wake up from this madness soon.

"Your obstacle and handicap, as you have stated, is your weight problem," he says. "To overcome this issue, the first step is to realize how important this goal is to you, which is now obvious since you listed it as a current Top Four Life Goal. The second step is to realize there is some work involved to learn the new habits. You can conquer most obstacles *with the right knowledge and the right perspective.* The goal of changing a deeply ingrained wrong mode of thinking is not an easy road. Once you give up the fantasy of *easily* changing your thinking about food and eating—instead of using great effort and tenacious attention—you can begin to conquer this beast."

I have read oodles of books on weight loss, and they are always about calories and exercise. This is poppycock and hooey.

"Let us talk about if you are willing to do the work of relearning how to think about food in this program. Can you imagine an NBA player saying 'I like basketball, but I do not want to spend time working out with weights and doing sprints'? There are unpleasant tasks that go with every goal. Champions do the work because *they want the goal.* You do the hard stuff because you want the good stuff."

I have been looking for a way to have the good stuff without embracing the hard stuff for years. Surely, somewhere, there is still a way.

"Do you think the great business owners got there because they played golf three days a week? No! *Great results are from great effort.* Until you hang up that fantasy of losing weight without effort, you are going to fail, because relearning how to eat and plan and shop and prep and do all that is coming, is definitely work. Elite Champions do not look for easy paths; they look for solutions and are willing to do the work and sacrifice."

It feels like this Genie is saying the same thing over and over again. He must think I am a slow learner. Maybe I should let him know I tied for valedictorian of my high school.

"Champions take the time to figure out what is needed, carve the time to do it, set margins so they will have energy to accomplish their top goals, and then give up lesser goals—playing pool, watching romcoms, painting, learning French, etcetera—for *that which they want most,* whether it is attending medical school, being an Olympic athlete, running an extraordinary business, or learning the lessons of *Skinny School.*"

I don't play pool—I can give up painting and learning French—but I don't think I can give up movies. I've seen *You've Got Mail* eight times.

"*Skinny School* will teach you to withstand key lime pie for the prize of size four jeans. Champions learn how to say no to their lower natures that want ease and comfort *right now.* Instead, Champions do what they need to do *in order to reach their true goals.* I will teach you to think like this."

Withstand key lime pie? I don't think he knows who he is dealing with.

"I will continually hound you about your desire for this goal to be effortless. I will not allow self-pity," he continues his rampage. "I will constantly admonish you for wanting things without paying the price. Yes, I will teach you how to eat, how to think, how to plan, how to shop, and how to navigate every temptation and situation. And if you follow my instructions, you will eventually reap the joy and elation of living in a thin body for your short time here on earth. *But it is work to learn it.* Deciding to pay the price to learn my *Skinny School* lessons is the difference between joyously romping through life as a skinny flip of a thing and fighting a lifelong battle with a ball and chain, aka excess weight."

This all sounds sort of loopy. I hope his secrets are not hypnotism or anything New Agey like that. Definitely, I'm not into that.

"It is time to give up looking for a magic pill to fix your problem, Young Jackie. Put on a mind-set that you have to pay a price for your goals. You will have to make choices, giving up some good things *to get the best things.* I have helped many women like you understand how they are thinking in a wrong manner and how to change their thoughts to accomplish long-term skinniness and emotional freedom from overeating."

He is a Genie. Why can I not get a dang magic pill?

"Valiant goals require valiant effort," he says.

This is melodramatic and far-fetched. I think of valiant goals like our American soldiers defending our country. Or I think of valiant goals like single mothers working three jobs to support their children. I do not think of weight loss in any heroic category like that. But, aside from his tendency to exaggerate, I do hear what he is saying. If I truly care about this goal, I will spend the time and effort to learn what he has to teach me, instead of continuing to do what I am doing now—*which is obviously not working.*

"Today's introduction may not seem like the traditional weight loss information," he says, "but in truth, until you give up looking for an easy path to get skinny and instead embrace the truth that diligent effort, time, sacrifice, and work will be required for relearning how to think about food, you will not succeed. You must *prioritize learning this material* in your life right now."

Is he going to lock me up and slip lettuce under the jail door?

"Young Jackie, this is where your weight loss struggle changes. You quit whining and complaining that conquering your problem is hard. Of course it is hard. If it was not, everybody would be skinny. Quit focusing on what you have to give up and focus on doing the assignments and work I am going to give you. Give up self-pity and take responsibility for whatever is necessary to succeed. Decide you will pay the price for being thin—because you really, truly care."

Oh…if only I could buy skinniness with one click on Amazon. Anyhow, this Genie has got me worried. This is a little creepy and scary, all this big talk about huge goals, elite Champion thinking, and so on. I just want to lose some weight. Why do I need all these excessive and inflated lectures? I feel like I should say a Pledge of Allegiance to weight loss.

The Genie continues, "Sometimes women will say to me, 'I do not have much time and energy for a bunch of lessons. Just give me a diet and a workout plan.' That is fine, but then I say, 'I cannot help you.' These women, though, are still struggling with their weight five years later. The reason is because there is a *deep-rooted thinking about food* that must be unearthed and retaught in order for me to help. No diet or workout can do that. People use food for entertainment and self-soothing, whereas food's primary function is fueling the body with nutrient-dense food when hungry. We have much to learn."

I don't want to learn something new. I want ease and comfort and I want it now. For example, a cupcake right now would be nice.

"*Skinny School* cannot be a little extra activity while you bustle around your overloaded life and then, *if you have time*, work on your *Skinny School* assignments. If you do that, you will just stay in your old, unsuccessful, frumpy patterns."

Oooh, there is that word I hate: *frumpy*.

Okay, enough niceness. Time for me to spout out my true objections. "Genie, I just *love* junk food. That is my problem." There. I said it. I love junk food. Deal with it, Genie.

"You humans eat illegitimate junk food all the time because you 'love' immediate gratification, but you are not getting you what you truly want, thinness and health. You are bigger than this. You can learn to have delayed gratification in one area so as to acquire a benefit—skinniness—that *you truly, deeply care more about* in another. Humans do not get *everything* they want. You must choose what you *really* want and then forgo other things to get them. The lessons in *Skinny School* will teach you how to think like this."

I have one more objection to throw at him. This is a good one. I sit up straight, throw my shoulders back, and get a slight smile on my face. "Genie, isn't the focus of women to be on their inner beauty? I mean, this feels like a focus on outward beauty."

He pauses, which has been unusual so far for the Genie. He looks me squarely in the eye. "Of course, the priority of human women should be on their inner beauty. However, that does not negate the *importance and need for self-control* in eating and *for attaining knowledge* about healthy and wise eating." He continues to stare at me.

I guess he shot my holier-than-thou statement down. Oh well, it was worth a try.

"For a woman to decide once and for all that she cares more about permanent thinness than an immediate food sensation is the one huge decision she has to make. You have tasted it all, you have tried eating it all, and it has not gotten you what you really want. Until you are ready to change how you *think*, no diet in the world can help you. Women who have learned to eat for nutrition and hunger instead of self-soothing and entertainment do not miss the junk food. Their enjoyment of their thin bodies is so outstanding and superior that they cannot believe they did not give up junk food years ago."

Yeah, that will be the day, when I can give up junk food. That likelihood is similar to J. Crew calling me and telling me they want me to be the model on the cover of their next catalog. I am even too chubby to be a plus-size model.

"Young Jackie, if thinness is really important and a woman is mentally prepared to work hard to acquire new habits and thinking, then she can truly be thin the rest of her life."

I have sort of felt like a victim in the past. He says I am in charge and responsible. Bummer.

"What you find in women who are thin—the ones that are *not* naturally thin—is that they have a mind-set of how they eat and how they exercise, and they even have rules for cheating. Food, they have learned, is not to be used to change how they feel; instead, they use food to build and nourish their bodies. These women want to live their lives in thin bodies, so that means they think a certain way, eat a certain way, move a certain way, every day, the rest of their lives. They do not go on a diet. They approach food with a mind-set that they will have to find another way to soothe and entertain themselves. Food is to nourish their bodies, albeit a delicious one. By choosing *what they eat, how much they eat, and how much they move their bodies*, wise women realize they have complete control over their weight…and they are happy about this."

Why can it not be true that a bag of Chips Ahoy speeds up the metabolism?

"Their mind-set of eating in a certain way and moving every day must be learned and embraced to such an extent that it *overrides* the previous deep grooves in the brain. It can be likened to learning to read and write Chinese. You cannot read a book over a weekend and then be able to read and write Chinese. *The sustained effort you give the program determines the extent to which you are able to override your previous wrong programming.*"

Sustained effort? I want a miracle, and I want it yesterday.

"Get clear on what you want and how long you have wanted it. Get clear on the fact that you are going to have to take major strides to overturn this deeply ingrained thinking habit. Deeply ingrained habits, like eating junk food, take at least six months to override. Commit now to working on Skinny School daily for that time segment."

No one says this. Not NBC. Not ABC. Not Fox. I truly believe Katie Couric would have heard this and reported on it if it were true.

"How many years have you wanted this? How much more would you enjoy your life if you were at your best weight? We are now going to create List Two in your Ruby Journal."

My thoughts wander as I pick up the jeweled journal and open to a clean page. Why do men have to prefer skinny chicks? Why can't a man's first choice be a woman who is forty-five pounds overweight?

"Entitle this page 'List Two: My Goal Weight,'" the Genie says. "Write down Goal A, which is what you would absolutely love to weigh. Then, write Goal B, a weight three pounds above that. And last, add two more pounds to Goal B, and that is your Scream Zone. You may have to later change these goals, but this will get you started."

I am five foot nine and have a small bone frame, so 130 pounds would be a good Goal A for me. That would make Goal B 133 pounds, with 135 being the Scream Zone. I write it all down.

"Young Jackie, I would like you to weigh *every morning* when you first get up. By weighing every day, you are forced to be objective about your progress. And even after you are at your Goal A weight, weighing every day is protection. When you hit your Scream Zone weight, you can take serious action before you regain fifteen or twenty pounds."

Again, stupid advice. Everyone now says throw away your scales and look in the mirror. This guy's advice is antiquated.

"One last thing," the Genie says. "You humans do better when you are operating in groups. It was the way you were designed. Find two to five other friends and reteach the material that I teach you. The best way for humans to learn anything is to teach it."

Oh, right. I can see me now asking my friends to let me teach them what a Genie taught me. Sure, that is believable.

"Genie, I am not sure my friends would…"

He cuts me off as if he knows what I am going to say. "Tell them you have a new weight loss coach and you want to share with them what you are learning. If they are suffering because of their weight, they will be interested."

I think of Beth and the weight she has gained since she has had a baby. I will think about sharing this information with her, but I am not promising anybody anything.

"You need to be patient with this program, Young Jackie. There is a 'click' and a 'flip' in women's brains around Lesson Seven, when they say, 'Oh, my gosh, I get this and I can do it for the rest of my life.' Around Lesson Seven, the pieces will all start fitting together, and you will be able to comprehend the whole *Skinny School* mentality. But you have to trust me, do the written exercises I give you, and work this program daily for a while before you get it. Agreed?"

I nod my head yes, but I cross my fingers behind my back because I am not sure at all if I am going to keep this promise. A Genie, a Ruby Journal, and some imbecilic secrets or lessons. Horse feathers.

"You have wanted this for thirteen years," he says. "This situation causes you more grief and discomfort than any other. You are going to learn to forego immediate gratification and choose delayed gratification because *that gets you what you really want: thinness*! I am going to Arabia to get a rubdown with some Dead Sea salts. I will return shortly. There is a recipe for Genie Meatballs in your fridge." And the Genie suddenly vanishes into thin air.

What? He is gone? No food charts? No lists? No exercise plans? Just a big talk about effort, goals, and retraining the brain? This is what I get when I ask to be skinny? A psychologist's babbling? I do not think he gets me or weight loss. I am pretty disgusted with this whole Genie thing. I get one wish, and then I get this soapbox twaddle?

This is the stupidest weight loss advice I have ever heard. Why can't he give me a boot camp exercise program and a diet with restricted calories? What is with all this mumbo jumbo with current Top Four Life Goals? This guy doesn't know what he is talking about, and I wasted my one wish. Dang. I should have asked for money.

Anyhow, what is he going to ask me to give up? I cannot live on celery and radishes. My food is very important to me. Why, it gives me predictable comfort and pleasure. What is going to replace that?

One thing I have to give the Genie in spite of all that balderdash is that I do feel a new awareness of *how much I care*. I mean, this *is* definitely in my current Top Four Life Goals. It is enlightening to hear myself say it. But I am to learn some idiotic secrets? Why cannot life be easy and fun filled, like a continual vacation at Atlantis in the Bahamas with poolside service from the restaurant?

Helping myself to a large bowl of ice cream, I decide to think about all of it later. I also get a few chocolate-chip cookies I have stashed in the pantry and crumble them on top of the ice cream. And…maybe a little chocolate syrup to top it all off. This will surely drown out the thoughts of what a loser I am. I head to my bedroom and get comfortable on my bed while I eat my treat. Like Scarlett O'Hara, I will think about all of this *tomorrow*.

My text message tone beeps, and it is from Beth: **Richard told me Zach hired you after only forty minutes! I knew they would love you! So what did you think of the boss's daughter, Eva? Definitely a downside to the job.**

Beth and I are always on the same page.

I begin to text back that Rachel is the Rachel of my high school nightmares, but there is a knock at the door. Oh! I forgot Robert said he was coming over. I had better hide this ice cream fast because Robert thinks I am on a diet. Sticking the ice cream under my bed, I get up to answer the door. Also, I must soon deal with how far Robert is from the man of my dreams.

The nonnegotiable in *Skinny School* so far is:

1. I expect to work hard like a Champion to retrain my mind since this is a current Top Four Life Goal.

Note to Reader: Please go back and reread the sentences you underlined and highlighted (remember, this is a workbook). Write the Genie's thoughts that especially speak to you in your Ruby Journal. All of the Ruby Journal lists are included in Appendix A at the back of this book.
Also, all of the Genie recipes can be found at JulieNGordon.com/ SkinnySchool.

Lesson 2

Sugar and Starches are NOT Your Friends

Wednesday, August 13   Weight: 177   Pounds gained: 2   Need to lose: 47

My weight was up two pounds this morning from yesterday's craziness and as usual, that spirals me into a funk. As I drive to Fortwright's office to start the day, my mind rehearses how to tell Mr. Fortwright I am quitting in two weeks. Every idea I have stinks.

My mind wanders to the meeting with the Genie yesterday and his grand presentation about goals, sacrifice, and making the effort to learn what really works in weight loss. Ridiculous. I know what works: a twelve-hundred-calorie diet (even though I have tried that for years). Anyhow, how ludicrous this whole thing is. I asked to be skinny, and the word *calorie* was never mentioned! Now that is pathetic.

At a stoplight, I glance at my reflection in the rearview mirror, and even my clear skin and white teeth do not cheer me up. My wide hips that spread out on the seat below me sink me lower into gloom. And on top of that, I have got to deal with this issue that I do not like my boyfriend.

Exhaling heavily, I feel very discouraged. What I am really upset about is that I am fat and I do not see any answers. Sure, I got a wish from the Genie, but I am pretty sure all his advice is baloney.

Spiraling down into despondency, I think of how I have been chubby for thirteen years. I have been the pretty-but-fat girl for a long time. My thoughts trail back to my first day as a junior in a new high school. Our family had just moved to Memphis a couple of weeks before and I knew no one. As I got out of my car in the school parking lot, a pickup truck full of muscled jocks drove by on the other side of my aisle, obviously only seeing me from the shoulders up. I heard one of them yell, "Dudes! Look at the new girl. She's hot. Wow." They all started hee-hawing, hooting, and driving back around so they would run into me, the hot new girl, in the parking lot.

Holding my head up high, I acted like I had no idea these popular, chiseled boys were on a mission to run into me. With regal dignity, I walked toward my new school.

When the jocks got to the row where they could see *all* of me, one of the boys yelled, "Gawd, she's fat!" and they drove off, punching each other and laughing hysterically.

Another similar instance I vividly remember was when I was pledging a sorority in college and the sorority sent around a sheet to the fraternity houses with head shots of its new pledges. Reggie Tyson saw my picture, called me up, and asked me out. For the next four days before our date, we spent hours on the phone, laughing, telling stories, teasing, and falling madly in crush. What anticipation I had as he texted me from the dorm lobby to say he was here to get me. I walked out into the lobby to meet Reggie. At first, he could only see me from the shoulders up as the front desk was blocking his full view. I almost detected love in his eyes. Love that wanted us to be a couple. Love that was ready to exclusively date. But the second I rounded the corner and he got a full-body view, his countenance fell in a nanosecond. I was home by 9:30 p.m. Reggie Tyson later told an older girl in the sorority that I had the best personality of any girl he had ever met. Imagine that—the best personality of any girl he had ever met, yet he brought me home at nine thirty. Boys just do not like fat girls.

I am twenty-eight now, and still solidly single (no pun intended). Every day of my life I get up and say that today is the day that I will become a skinny flip of a thing. And every night of my life, I go to bed and say that tomorrow is the day that I will become a skinny flip of a thing. The days when I am going to start tomorrow have run together, and now I have fought a weight problem for thirteen years. And even though I now have a Genie and a magic wish, I know exactly nothing about what to do about my problem. What a bummer this Genie guy is.

Fortwright gets to work around ten thirty, and I sorrowfully and gently give him my two weeks' notice. Actually, I think he is fighting back tears. He has become such a pitiful thing, all saggy-faced in his wrinkled khaki suit. I am sure the moist eyes are not as much about me as they are about his desperate drinking problem, compounded now by the fact that his first mate is jumping ship. Giving him the names and websites of two recovery centers, I hope he will realize how severe his situation is and enter treatment.

After a normal workday, I quickly drive home as Robert is picking me up in a few minutes so we can meet BFF Beth and her husband, Richard, for dinner. Although Robert and I have been dating for nine months, he still does not like to be with my friends. Occasionally, like tonight, he acquiesces. After listing my current Top Four Life Goals with the Genie yesterday, I get a queasy feeling every time I think about Robert and how he is not even close to my goal of marrying the man of my dreams. Robert always said he was a person of faith, but lately, I have questioned if his faith is authentic, since so many of this actions contradict those beliefs.

Taking a quick bath, I grab the sundress I laid out to wear and look for my gold sandals with the matching clutch purse. They were right here this morning. Immediately, I know where they are. I text Tory, my roommate. **Tory, I cannot find my gold sandals and purse. Would you happen to know where they are?**

She texts right back. **Oh, so so sorry!! ☹ I had no idea you were going to wear them tonight. So so sorry! ☹ I'll be back around 11:00 p.m.**

My annoyance is more than slight. I have asked her twice not to wear my things unless she asks first, and she has again ignored my request. Soon I must deal with the whole Tory/roommate situation, but right now, I have got to find some shoes to wear.

Throwing on some old flip-flops, I simmer with resentment at Tory. Borrowing my clothes is not Tory's only roommate sin. She is a month behind in paying her half of the rent.

Opening the fridge to get some juice while waiting on Robert, I notice there is leftover chocolate cake. Although I am going to dinner in a few minutes, a couple bites will not hurt, and it will calm me down from being upset over Tory. I eat two bites, then four bites, and in a couple of minutes, I have downed a large piece of chocolate cake, right before I am to head out to dinner. Oh my, I am so insane, insane, insane.

Robert arrives, and I drag my disgusted self out to his car to drive to the Brazilian Steakhouse. Robert begins his usual chatting, telling me about his day. When I first met Robert, he sort of swept me off my feet. On our first date, a limousine came to pick me up and drove us all over the city, like a progressive dinner party. We ate appetizers at the Palm restaurant, had the main dish at Capitol Grille, and then finished with dessert at Sperry's. Robert talked incessantly about his extensive travel and told long stories of people he had met. Initially, I was infatuated. But as time has gone on, I have wondered if any of the stories are even true. His wads of hundred-dollar bills are always crammed in his wallet. He says he works for his father, but I do not see how that small business would give Robert the kind of cash he consistently throws around.

Three months ago we bought a ski boat together. I am still not quite sure how he talked me into this, but I paid half. Robert did not seem to mind my weight at first, and I was therefore comfortable in a bathing suit in front of him, which is incredibly unusual for me. Robert and I have spent most Saturdays this past summer waterskiing at the lake. I do love waterskiing, and Robert was someone who liked overweight me. The beauty and serenity of the sun and the lake made me blind and indifferent to what a braggart and bore Robert really is.

As I said, for the first few months, Robert was accepting of my weight. But a couple weeks ago, we were with some of his friends at the Nashville Sounds baseball game, and afterward, the group went to get ice cream. I ordered one scoop of butter pecan topped with another scoop of blueberry. In front of his friends, Robert said, "Jackie is on a diet. When she is on a diet, she orders two scoops of ice cream instead of her usual three." His friends thought it was hilarious. I was completely humiliated. Why, Robert's acceptance of my weight was one of the main things I expected from him. When I confronted him later, he pleaded innocent and promised never to do it again. Actually, I have not forgotten or forgiven that moment.

Repeatedly, I have told myself Robert is the best I can do. I mean, I do not want to be alone forever, and I cannot seem to attract the kind of guy I really want.

Upon arriving at the Brazilian Steakhouse, Robert and I join Beth and Richard, who are seated on the far side of the restaurant. Even before the server approaches our table, Robert is off on a long story, which no one feels they can interrupt: "So the guy behind me in the bank line then said…" The server has to stand and wait for an extended period of time, so Robert can find a place to pause the story long enough for us to give our drink order.

Frankly, I am embarrassed. Beth and Richard act as if they are not annoyed at all. They love me, and if Robert is my boyfriend, then he gets a pass.

Usually I am careful not to eat too much in front of others (I do the real damage alone). The large piece of chocolate cake I ate before dinner does take the edge off my appetite, and I don't really get to enjoy the crab cakes, baked potato, bread, and cheesecake the way I usually do. But I eat it all anyway.

The whole night, Robert monopolizes the conversation. Again, I think of the Top Four Life Goals exercise I did with the Genie. Marrying the man of my dreams is certainly a joke when I think about marrying Robert.

Back in his car after dinner, Robert begins another long story about his great-great-grandfather and his servants on their plantation. Suddenly, I decide I cannot throw off Robert's incessant and boring bragging/storytelling any longer. I cannot take one more second of this. Not one. Fat or not, I would rather be alone than be forced to listen to one more story. I want free from this backpack of bricks.

"Robert, I think we might need to take a break," I cowardly say, knowing I should tell him I am axing him forever.

"Really, Jackie? Why? What is wrong? We can fix things," he says. Of course, Robert wants to talk about it, understand it, comb through every nuance and try to see if there is any way we can salvage this relationship. When one person wants to move on, the left-behind person invariably reacts this way.

"You can have my share of the boat, by the way," I say. That is around two thousand dollars, but hey, when you want to cut relationship ropes, you want to cut them *now*, money or no money.

Realizing how serious I am about the breakup when I willingly give up my share of the boat, Robert cannot wait to get me out of the car. I hear him mutter, "Good riddance to you and your fat…" His voice trails off as he speeds off with screeching tires. I could not exactly hear the last word, but I have a pretty good idea what it was.

I am stunned. Really stunned. Surely he did not just say that. He wouldn't, would he? But yes, he did. I want to kick him. I want to throw cold water in his face. I want to puncture his tires. The nerve of that rude, bragging, boring idiot.

My anger intensifies as I watch Robert drive off, realizing his character is even lower than I thought. Despair mixes with anger as I contemplate the wasted months I spent with him. Here I am, alone in a parking lot, being insulted by a loser ex-boyfriend. How does this happen to me? How do I always return to this square, a fat girl, alone? How will this ever be any different? I will never be able to date who I want.

Thoughts of Zach Boltz's upright, disciplined work ethic, his self-controlled speech, and his outrageous intense olive-green eyes erupt in my mind. I quickly banish those thoughts, knowing that I could never date a Zach-type. Those guys are reserved for the snooty Rachels of the world.

"Let us go inside and we will have Lesson Two, Young Jackie," a voice behind me says. **I am startled at first but quickly realize it is the Genie**. Between quitting my job today, having severe roommate issues, being humiliated by Robert, and now, a Genie appearing in my life, I feel I might crack up.

"I broke up with my loser boyfriend tonight because of your Top Four Life Goals exercise," I say.

"Bravo," he says, in a chirpy mood. Even though my nerves are twisted into a wad, my mood begins to soothe, just being in the presence of this up-beat sage. "Getting in touch with what is really important in your life helps streamline your decisions and makes you go after what you truly want. I am proud of you, Young Jackie. Tonight, we are going to discuss Lesson Two in *Skinny School*: Sugar and Starches are NOT your Friends."[2]

Sugar is definitely my friend, as well as my main consoler, so I do not know what he is talking about. Anyhow, after the earthquakes of today, I would rather not listen to a lecture but instead get a few cookies and go to bed.

"Tonight I will present information to you that all the new science sup-ports," he says. "It is what I have known and taught for centuries."

This guy looks like he is ready for a St. Patrick's Day parade but thinks he is a scientist. Sure.

"There are four different aspects to this lesson," he says. "One, we will discuss how hormones primarily drive weight loss or weight gain. Two, and of ultimate importance, I will teach you how to get rid of those incessant and demanding cravings that you now cannot resist. Three, we will talk about how sugar and junk food derail your long-term health. And topic number four will be the astounding and marvelous food you get to eat in *Skinny School*."

Speaking of fab food, I think there is still some chocolate cake in the fridge.

"The first subject we will discuss in our lesson tonight is what really drives weight loss or weight gain: your *hormones*. Listen well, Young Jackie, because here is the money: *certain foods cause certain hormones to be released*. So in es-sence, *by choosing* what *you eat*, you tell hormones whether to store fat or burn fat."

Why have I not heard about this hormone mumbo jumbo before? I watch TV, and Jimmy Kimmel never mentions it.

"This teaching is not complicated," he says. "Starches and sweets turn on hormones that tell your body *to store fat*. Therefore, if you *ditch starches and*

---

2   I am a counselor/coach whose goal is to change the way you *think* about food and eating. Therefore, since I am not a doctor or a nutritionist, I have listed my favorite health gurus in Appendix D. I suggest you read more of their amazing materials.

sweets and replace them with proteins, good fats, and vegetables, you overhaul your metabolism and switch it into a fat-burning mode."

Ditch starches and sweets? How ridiculous. Those are my two favorite kinds of food.

"Your culture has accepted that it is their birthright to have daily, delicious sugary and starchy foods," he says. "Desserts are deemed essential, expected, and revered in your circles. However, experts are now saying that we should not eat more than *fifteen to twenty grams of sugar a day* for weight loss. Have you checked the sugar on the strawberry yogurt you ate this morning? It has twenty-six grams of sugar in a single serving. The large piece of chocolate cake that you ate before dinner had thirty-nine grams of sugar. And the soda you had at the restaurant had forty grams of sugar. That is one hundred and thirty grams of sugar, and that is only about half of what you ate today."

Uhhh…half of the sugar I ate today? So I am eating over two hundred and fifty grams of sugar, and I am supposed to eat a mere twenty grams? Doesn't he realize I am a mere mortal?

"Another issue you must confront, Young Jackie, is that simple and refined carbs metabolize into sugar and therefore also produce hormones that signal your body to store fat."

No, no, he is not going to try to take away my chips, bread, pasta, pancakes, bagels, rolls, croutons, and crackers, is he? Please, no.

"The second topic that I want to discuss is how to get rid of those irresistible cravings you nightly experience," he says. "Are you ready for some shocking news? You are addicted to sugar. Yes, addicted, like a drug user. Your brain now releases dopamine that insists you eat, or otherwise, you feel like you might die.

Every night I fall under a spell in which no longer I, but food, is in control. It is as though I enter a trance and go unconscious.

"Cravings are urgent, demanding, and intense," he continues. "You cannot reason with them any more than you can reason with a hungry shark. They win. No contest. They hijack your brain. Cravings begin to peak, feel powerful and majestic, like the emperor of the world has spoken, and you, the weakling, must obey. This huge force is merely a craving, caused by an addiction to sugar. You have to get off sugar and refined carbs to get rid of the cravings."

No, no. I cannot get off sugar and carbs. I can't. I just can't.

"You cannot out-choose the beast of sugar addiction," he says. "It is a drug, and it is too strong. You must get rid of the craving by getting rid of the monster of too much sugar in your diet."

Sugar is not a monster. Sugar is delight, pleasure, and escape.

"When you get almost all of the sugar and starches out of your body, the cravings will leave. You will never overcome those intense cravings while allowing abundant sugar in your diet."

I would like to argue, but I must agree that every evening, my brain gets hijacked, and I end up eating what I pledge in the morning I won't. This has been going on for, eh, around thirteen years.

"Giving up sweets and simple starches will free you from your physical cravings," he says. "This is the number one thing with which women with weight loss issues struggle: *the willingness* to give up sweets and simple starches."

Well, duh. Sweets and starches are my entertainment, my stimulation, and my self-soothing mechanisms. How does he expect me to give up all that?

"Genie, if I am addicted, then how do I get off sweets and starches?" I ask incredulously, thinking that there is no way I could give up those two lovelies.

"You start eating *good food,* that is how," he says. "Many *Skinny School* graduates say they experience almost flu-like symptoms for a few days as their bodies begin to detoxify. But these same women then say they regain their sanity and their emotional equilibrium after they wean themselves from sugar and refined carbs."

I had no idea that I was *addicted* to sugar. Surely he is wrong about this. Me? Addicted? Naw...

"Imagine you were a mother and had a child that came home from school every day at three thirty, and every day, a bully was hiding in the same bushes. This bully jumped out, punched your kid, and ran away. What if it happened every day and you ignored it?"

"Genie, that would never happen. When I become a mother someday, I am going to take incredible care of my children."

"I am sure you will, Young Jackie. But this analogy is to explain what happens to you every day as far as your eating goes. You are addicted to sugar, and every day, the uncontrollable cravings come to taunt you. Daily, they punch you and beat you up. Yet you have refused to deal with the sugar and refined carbs that are driving the cravings. You cannot get rid of the bully of cravings until you get rid of sugar and refined carbs."

Is it possible that my love affair with sugar and refined carbs needs to be confronted? Oh my, this can't be true.

"There will be no success until you deal with the sugar and refined carb issue," he strongly states again. "If you continue to eat them, you will continue to have cravings. The dopamine in a sugar addict's brain is similar to the dopamine in a cocaine addict's brain."

Again, what he is saying is bizarre. He is comparing me to a dope addict.

"Giving up sweets and starches is known in many circles as 'eating clean,'" he says. "I will help you learn to do this, but you must understand you cannot move forward in *Skinny School* until this principle is embraced."

How ridiculously radical he is about this sweet/starch junk. I will have to think about it.

"That brings us to subject three for tonight, which is that excessive sweets and junk food *are harmful to your long-term health*. The culture has a gigantic blind spot and thinks that refined carbs and sugar are innocent and neutral to your health," he says. "They are anything but innocent and neutral. Food with a lot of sugar should have a skull-and-crossbones warning on it."

This is preposterous. I must challenge him on this. "Genie, fruit has sugar in it. Should fruit have a skull and crossbones on it?" That should get him. Maybe he needs to bring in another Genie who is a *real* expert in this area.

"Of course, fruit is a marvelous natural food," he says. "And scrumptious fruit is loaded with phytonutrients and antioxidants. However, for centuries, there was no refrigeration and no modern mass transportation, so fruit was therefore only available seasonally. And add to that, fruit has been bred to make it ultra sweet. Many Americans now consume too much fruit, since to lose weight, people need to watch their sugar grams."

No one says to watch your fruit intake. Why, on many programs, fruit is unlimited. This advice is outlandish. This guy could be sued for malpractice with this advice.

"I know you are mainly interested in weight loss, Young Jackie, but it is important to acknowledge that excessive sugar and refined carbs are bad for your long-term health. Your body was created to eat protein, good fats, vegetables, nuts, and seeds."[3]

"You are committing slow suicide when you eat all the sweets and refined carbs that you eat," he continues. "You would not put molasses in your car's gas tank, but yet you put substances in your one and only body all day long that your body was never designed to handle."

I still don't believe there is anything wrong with sugar and refined carbs. Would not the government protect us and make sure we did not eat harmful substances?

"I am going to introduce you to the term *Trash Food*. Trash Food is anything that does not promote your health and your ideal weight. Trash Food is the food that messes up your life by messing up your metabolism and health. People call cake, pie, and candy *treats*. Those foods are actually Trash Foods. After you reach your goal weight, you can have a BLT—bite, lick, or taste—but Trash Food keeps you addicted to sugar, produces hormones that signal your body to store fat, derails your optimum health goals, and ruins one of your current Top Four Life Goals of being thin. To acquire the dream of permanently living in your dream thin body, then this step is nonnegotiable."

Whoa, slow down there, buddy boy. You are calling those gorgeous concoctions Trash Food? I am not ready for this thinking. Not by a lonnng shot. I am pretty sure this idiotic *Skinny School* is not going to work for me. The magazines at the grocery store checkout offer diets that say you can eat anything you want. I would rather have those diets.

---

3 Dairy is highly debatable, and many people are intolerant to milk products. The reader will have to decide for herself about this issue.

"That brings me to our fourth and final subject of the day: *what you will eat.* By eating delicious and delectable food, you will see that my program is not one of huge deprivation. There is so much breathtaking and spectacular food to eat that my *Skinny School* students say they barely miss Trash Food at all."

Liar, liar, pants on fire. That is complete bunk.

"As you probably know, there is good nutrition in complex carbs," he says, "such as brown rice and sweet potatoes. And it is fine if you add back a few of those complex carbs *after* you lose all your weight. But for now, we are going to *eliminate* almost all starches and sugar from your diet, keeping your carb count to fifty grams a day and your sugar count to fifteen grams a day."

"What about Eva," I ask, "who eats sugar-loaded yogurt, tons of fruit, bagels, and candy bars? She is a stick, Genie."

"Eva has a very high metabolism," he says. "And although she is able to remain thin, her diet is not healthy because of the large amount of sugar she eats."

I wonder how much sugar was in that whole bag of Oreos that I downed last week.

"You now believe many lies, Young Jackie. One of them is 'Trash Food is desirable.' You also believe that 'Trash Food is neutral toward my health.' Both of those sentences are lies."

Trash Food, as he calls it, is desirable, even if he says it is not. His so-called Trash Food is mind-blowing and marvelous.

"Gorgeous and delicious food is one of the most fabulous pleasures on earth," he says. "You will learn the delight of *healthy* food. Examples would include quiche—no crust—free-range fried chicken made with almond flour, nitrate-free bacon and cage-free eggs, salads with goat cheese and Caesar dressing, grass-fed steak, wild-caught lobster and shrimp, nuts, free-range roasted chicken, almond-sautéed green beans, omelets, luscious sauces for veggies, broccoli cheese soup, bacon cheeseburgers, and so on. You still get to eat delicious food, just not delicious Trash Food."

All that food does sound yummy.

"Focus on all the beautiful food you get to eat, *not on the food you cannot eat,*" the Genie says.

I do like quiche and I love bacon cheeseburgers. I guess I could try his *Skinny School* principles for a little while. Of course, I can quit if I want.

"Your assignment is to begin to pay attention to how many grams of sugar and carbs you eat. Do not eat more than fifty carbs a day and no more than fifteen grams of sugar a day."

That is too restrictive. I don't think I can do that.

"Vegetables are the secret weapon in this program: they fill you up, make you healthy, and turn on the right hormones. Be sure to eat six or more servings a day and preferably eight to twelve servings. Add vegetables to every feeding."

A feeding? He is talking to me like I am a monkey at the zoo.

"Eat healthy proteins, such as grass-fed beef, natural chicken and turkey without antibiotics and hormones, pork that is raised with care, wild-caught fish, and cage-free eggs."[4]

You cannot buy that stuff at my local grocery store, can you? Now I have to drive to a health food store? This is way too much work.

"Add some raw nuts and seeds, a little fruit (since sugar grams add up fast), some good fats such as avocados, coconuts, olive oil, nuts, grass-fed meat, and butter made from raw, grass-fed organic milk, and some dairy, such as cheese, if you can handle the lactose."

I wonder if ice cream is considered legitimate dairy.

"So, eh...what specific foods do I not eat?" That may sound like a stupid question, but I like exact instructions.

"Do not eat starches, such as bread, pasta, crackers, croutons, potatoes, chips, tortillas, flour, pizza, or pancakes. And do not eat sweets, such as candy, sodas, cakes, pies, or doughnuts. All these foods tell your hormones to quit burning fat and store it instead."

Oh, dear. Surely there is a plan somewhere that still lets me eat all my favorite foods. But to be honest, I have tried a hundred of them, and I have never had any long-term success so far.

---

4 As you may recognize, this food plan is very similar to many Paleo diets.

"It is true that some women can have a dessert every day and still be thin," he says. "One of three things is going on in that scenario. One, they are naturally thin and have a very high metabolism. Two, they are exercising a huge amount. Or three, they are meticulously watching their entire caloric intake and are not eating much at their other feedings. The healthiest thing to do is to not eat Trash Food at all. And definitely *with your compulsive eating style* and your *addiction to sugar*, you personally need to get rid of Trash Food altogether."

"So Genie," I ask, shocked by this horrible news, "does that mean I will never have a cookie again?"

"Later in the program, Lesson Twenty-Two, I will introduce the concept of Planned Cheating, which will include a very small amount of festivity eating. It will be planned and controlled, so the answer to your question is that you will be able to eat a cookie again, but it will never be the same as now, when you eat in a sporadic, unplanned, or overindulgent way."

I do not love that answer, but at least it seems more reasonable than telling me that I will never eat anything sweet again.

"Again, many women wrongly think they are entitled to be thin *and* to also eat whatever they want," he says. "Until women learn to give up the pleasure and comfort of Trash Food—that is, sugar and starches—for a higher pleasure, thinness, they will be stuck in the overweight and despair cycle. The day your long-term weight loss begins to happen is the day you realize you cannot have both, eating whatever and whenever you want, *and still being thin.*"

Forever? Forever is a long time. I can do this for a while, but I am not giving up sugar and grains forever.

"It is time to take the mask off Trash Food," he says. "Sugar and refined carbs are *not* your friends. They are masquerading as your friends, offering temporary comfort and entertainment, but in reality, they are traitors that keep you from one of your current Top Four Life Goals, thinness and health."

A mask? Traitors? He is calling all that yummy food that I have cuddled up with for years those names? This is going to take some time to get used to.

"I want to be crystal clear about this one more time, Young Jackie. Women try and try to have both—that is, they try to keep sugar and starches in their diet and also to be thin. The sugar and simple starches in a woman's diet keeps her addicted to sugar, and therefore, she will continue to have cravings, which she is not able to resist. She must put down a stake and say that she will find pleasure in all the fabulous, legitimate food available. Women who give up sweets and simple carbs revel in delight over their newfound emotional stability as well as their narrow hips. This is not a plan of deprivation, but a plan of freedom, freedom from all the despair, discouragement, and self-disgust that have reigned in your life because *of a reluctance to deal with the sugar and starches in your life.* You cannot go on with *Skinny School* until you embrace this lesson. The other lessons will be in vain."

Maybe he is just blowing smoke. Maybe I can keep a few extra sugars and starches and still lose weight. Maybe he is just worked up and carrying on tonight, and in our next meeting, he will calm down and consider letting me have more sweets. I mean, wouldn't my church talk about this if sugar and simple starches were so bad? Why, they have donuts out every Sunday!

"Start tracking and logging your sugar and carb grams. There are many free apps and websites available to help you track these, such as MyFitnessPal. You will not always have to track your sugar and carbs the rest of your life, but it is necessary for now so you can learn the sugar and carb gram counts of foods. Also, apps like MyFitnessPal track calories. We are not as concerned about calories right now as we are sugar and carb grams. However, calories *do matter*, and some foods that have no sugar or carb grams, like nuts and sausage, are actually full of calories, so you need to go easy on those foods. Watching the calories on MyFitnessPal add up daily will be good feedback for you. But for now, the focus will be on lowering your sugar and carb totals. Remember, *the way to give up Trash Food is to focus on eating good food.* I have to get a massage in Venezuela. I have left Genie Taco Salad in your fridge."

He disappears, and I feel helpless. He still did not give me an exact plan, in my opinion. I just got a bunch of general principles. Eek! "Genie!" I yell, but it does no good. He might be my Genie, but he comes and goes on his own schedule. They do not make Genies like they used to.

Walking toward my apartment door, I dig in my purse to find the key. This whole new concept of certain foods turning on hormones that determine if my body stores or burns fat is colossal. And the whole concept that sugar and refined carbs are the culprits that are driving my cravings is blowing my mind. This new paradigm is outrageous. Could it be true? Is my old way of thinking about food and eating all wrong? I am going to need a lot more convincing than this. Surely a lot of what he said is wrong.

Also, I am severely annoyed that I ask to be skinny and then I get a dissertation on work ethic and sacrifice, and then a royal condemnation of sugar! Geez. Again, where is my exercise program and twelve-hundred-calorie plan?

Opening the door to the apartment, I notice the kitchen is a colossal mess. There are pans, bowls, and measuring cups all over the kitchen. On the counter is a sticky note that says, SORRY ABOUT THE MESS. ☹ L I WILL GET IT CLEANED UP IN THE MORNING. TORY.

Tory, my roommate who does not pay rent, borrows my things without asking and leaves her huge pile of dirty dishes in the kitchen. Another issue to deal with soon.

I consider texting my sister, Jessica, in Memphis. Since she is a night owl, I bet she is up. There are four girls in our family. Allison is the oldest, Jessica is next, and then there's Chloe. I was what you call the proverbial surprise years later. The three of them are thick as thieves. They call themselves the Three Memphis Musketeers. They tell me that if I move back to Memphis, we can be the Fantastic Four. I moved away from Memphis on purpose to get away from all the family drama, but I do miss Jess. Mom always said we were clones, only ten years apart.

The need to talk to someone who will understand about Loser Robert seems very important right now. So I text Jessica: **My life is horrible. Are you up?**

Ten seconds after I hit SEND, my cell rings.

Barely into my meltdown about Rude Robert, Jessica interrupts. "I am so glad you got rid of him. He was a terrible choice for you, Jackie. I have been waiting for this moment because Matthew"—her husband—"has a single client in Nashville that he wants to fix you up with."

Oh, no. Not a blind date. It is ridiculous how many times I have been sold to men as "pretty and witty," and then when they've seen my size, they've never called back. No. No. I am not going to be subjected to that again.

"Thanks, but no thanks, Jess. I really can't go, and I do not have anything to wear and—"

"Nonsense," she says, as she interrupts again. "Matthew and the boys are going camping Saturday, so I am free all day. I will drive to Nashville and be there by 10:00 a.m. Then we will find you the perfect outfit. Also I will tell Matthew to call Brandon and tell him you are free Saturday night."

You have to know my sister Jessica to understand why I acquiesced. She is a little persistent. Anyhow, what is one more night of humiliation in the scheme of life?

As soon as we hang up, I get another text message. It is probably from Robert, apologizing for his rude remark. No, it is from Mr. Fortwright.

I found a replacement for you (well, as if anyone could ever replace you, Jackie.) She will be here in the morning. Could you please train her tomorrow and Friday and let her start Monday?

Actually, that is good news because Zach wanted me to start as soon as possible. I will e-mail Zach tomorrow and let him know I will start working for him on Monday.

How am I supposed to ditch starches and sweets with all the turmoil I have in my life? And anyhow, what am I supposed to eat? He did not give me any recipes. I cannot live on broiled chicken and broccoli. This Genie guy better have some more helpful information soon, or I am asking for a replacement wish.

I want some Trash Food!

The nonnegotiables in *Skinny School* so far are:

1. I expect to work like a Champion to retrain my mind since this is a current *Top Four Life Goal*.
2. Ditching sweets and starches is not optional if I want to overhaul my metabolism. I am to track my sugar/carb grams as well as my calories. I focus on all the beautiful, delicious food *I get to eat* instead of what I must not eat.

Lesson 3

Preparation Is the Secret of Champions

Saturday, August 16   *Weight: 177*   *Pounds gained: 2*   *Need to lose: 47*

Jessica drove in from Memphis this morning and we went to Dillards. Really I would rather shop in boutique-type stores—Anthropologie, White House/ Black Market, J. Crew—but they do not carry tub sizes. Jessica might have missed her calling in life as a personal shopper. She found the most slimming gray slacks and a great-looking white tunic with a gray-and-turquoise scarf. After she did her magic on me, I looked ten pounds thinner. And before she drove back to Memphis, she insisted we get mani-pedis together. Since our mom was killed in a car wreck four years ago, Jessica has ramped up her older sister role.

Brandon will be here in a few minutes. I am so nervous, I am perspiring. At least my hair and makeup look good. I check the mirror. Ugh! I am such a fattie! Why did I agree to this blind date? This guy will not want to go out with a fat chick, and he—

Ding dong.

Oh, dear, he's here. No escaping now. I open the door.

"Hey, Jessica. I'm a couple minutes early. I hope that is all right."

This is my date? This old guy? Maybe this is the father of my date. This guy looks like he is almost fifty. What is going on?

"Brandon?" I ask. Surely this is the chauffeur.

"That's me. Do you want me to wait in the car since I am early?" he says. Trying to recover from the shock of this guy's age, I notice he is not bad looking. He has a decent build, is around six feet tall, has nice features and hair that is thinning a little around his crown—but hey, he is my dad's age!

"No, come in. Let me get my purse, and I am ready to leave."

Walking to my bedroom to get my purse, I quickly text Jessica: **You did not tell me that my date would have a walker.**

She texts back: **You would not have gone if you had known how old he was. Matthew says he has got a fabulous job and that he is a great guy. Give him a chance.**

I write, **Let's just hope he does not take his dentures out and put them in his water while we are eating.**

Jessica: **Give him a chance, will you? He is only forty-eight.**

Me: **You conveniently forgot to tell me that.** I start to write, **I am not this hard up,** but the truth is, I am.

We walk to his Porsche and begin our drive to Prime 108 restaurant. Brandon is very polite and a good conversationalist. He understands the dance of asking the right amount of questions and talking about himself a little, too. His cologne is a little strong, but old men often wear too much. His clothes have a classy, Brooks Brothers look.

Arriving at the restaurant, we are quickly seated. I order in a manner that would please the Genie: shrimp cocktail for an appetizer, a salad with oil and vinegar, a piece of broiled flounder with asparagus, and sautéed mushrooms in place of the potato. But I feel frustrated that I still do not know *exactly* what to eat. That should be the first thing we talk about with a diet! I still feel somewhat in the dark about this new eating plan.

Pulling my mind back to my date, I realize Brandon is actually kind of witty and obviously intelligent. However, I'm not sure I can handle this age difference. At least I don't see a hearing aid, so that is good.

Excusing myself to go to the bathroom, I again text Jessica: **Thank goodness he did not wear a cardigan.**

Jessica texts back: **Just give him a CHANCE, will you?**

I am about to leave the restroom and go back to my old-timer when I almost knock down the girl coming in. "Excuse me," she says and walks by without looking at me. I do not get a very good look at her, but something about her makes me look again. Now I have lived in Nashville four years, and I have never run into Rachel Hanover. And here we are, with me getting ready to work for Zach, and I run into her. An old fossil for a date and a ghost from my past, all in one night.

Rachel's light blue sundress shows off her tanned, sculpted shoulders. She is as tiny as she was in high school. The hem is an appropriate one inch above her skinny knees. Classy. Of course, this is what Zach would date. The Miss Tennessee type. Her skin is as beautiful as ever, but her eyes still bug out, if you ask me. The thought that she and Zach will see me with my grandfatherly date makes me upset. I decide not to speak and instead sneak out. But it is too late. She has seen me looking at her.

"Jackie? Is that you? Why, Zach told me he hired you. That is so funny! After all these years, you are working for Zach! I told him how smart you are."

Yeah, and I bet you told him how fat I was in high school, too, didn't you? Her friendliness is obviously the result of me working for her future husband. I have not forgiven how she ignored me in high school, or how she laughed at the "more time to eat banana splits" joke. I will have to work through that.

"Hi, Rachel. Nice to see you," I lie. "Yes, I am working for Zach. Is that not crazy?" A stupid thing to say, but I could not think of anything else. I wish I could hide. And I definitely want to hide Gramps.

We chat a little more and then, in a soft voice, Rachel says, "Oh, Jackie?"

She wants to say something else. Maybe she wants to have lunch now that I am working for Zach. Or maybe now she wants to be friends. Maybe she wants to apologize and say, "Let's let bygones be bygones."

I turn to her with an open heart. "Yes?"

"You have toilet paper under your foot," she says.

Humiliated to the core, I remove it and thank her.

Returning to the table, I notice that Gramps is texting. Most old guys are afraid of technology, so this is a good sign.

Really, I am being a little hard on Brandon. Why, he is very pleasant. Ten years older would be sexy, but I do not know if I can handle twenty. Again, Brandon asks questions and listens. He works internationally, and he drops names of cities that he visits, like Dubai, Istanbul, and Singapore. That life would sure beat the heck out of going to the lake every weekend with Robert.

I begin to tell Brandon a little about my crazy family when Zach walks up to our table. My gosh, the presence of Zach throws me for a loop. My insides flinch. Is it Josh Duhamel? Christian Bale? No, it is my future boss with his movie-star good looks. *Pull yourself together, Jackie,* I tell myself. Zach is the same low-key friendly that he was in the office as he shakes Brandon's hand. I bet he wants to know if I am eating with my father.

Zach Boltz. Now *that* is some catch. And little drill team captain Rachel Hanover threw out the bait and reeled him in. No surprise, really. That is the way it works. She is dating the equivalent of *The Bachelor*, and I am dating a baby boomer.

After dinner, Brandon and I arrive back at my apartment, and Tory is there. Usually when Robert used to come in, Tory would excuse herself to her bedroom. But tonight, she plops down on the sofa and decides to chat with us. My, oh my, she is *very* friendly. I mean, I do not care, because I do not particularly like Grandpa, but it still feels disrespectful to have your room-mate flirting with your date. Brandon is not acting overly interested in her, so that helps.

Trying hard not to let Brandon see me yawning, I fail. He says it is time for him to head home. "Early to bed, early to rise," he says, quoting Benjamin Franklin. Well, actually, he and Ben are about the same age, so no wonder he is quoting him.

Just before Brandon gets in his car, he asks me if I would like to go to the Train concert next weekend. He says he has tickets on the ninth row.

Ninth row? I LOVE Train.

"Train?" I ask. "This is not a drive-by, I, I, I, I..." I sing and do a little dance. Brandon smiles approvingly. I can tell he thinks I am cute, even though I am a tank.

I thought this would be our last date, but I decide I cannot say no to that request. Ninth-row seats rock.

"And Bon Jovi is coming to Nashville next month. I already have tickets and hope you will go with me then, too. My tickets to that concert are on the twelfth row."

Uh, did he say twelfth row? Bon Jovi? Those tickets probably cost around five hundred dollars apiece. Maybe this is not our last date after all. Train and Bon Jovi? Maybe I could get use to his gray hair and wrinkles.

We say goodnight and he leaves.

Moseying back to my bedroom, I take off my makeup, get under the covers, and turn off the light.

"You made some good choices at dinner tonight," I hear a voice say in the dark.

You would think I would be petrified, **but I immediately recognize the Genie's voice.** He switches on the lamp and hands me my Ruby Journal and a beautiful pen.

"And do not worry, no one can hear my voice except you," he says. "Tonight we will have Lesson Three, Preparation Is the Secret of Champions. These secrets will increase your daily Willpower Points," he says.

"Willpower Points?" I ask. More new cockamamie terms.

"Willpower Points are the combined forces you possess to make right choices and refuse unprofitable ones. Being tired will reduce your ability to choose well, as will being stressed, overly busy, and other situations such as these," he says.

Now *that* would be a multimillion-dollar business, if I could bottle and sell Willpower Points.

"As a human, you only have a finite amount of Willpower Points each day to spend," he continues. "Learning how to increase your Willpower Points each day will be one of your tickets out of the overweight dungeon you have been captive in. Your finite set of daily Willpower Points is diminished by arguing, being drained by a boring job, or having negative confrontations. When your Willpower Points are low, you will not have the same reserve to choose the right foods to eat."

I wonder if jealousy over the boss's mean toothpick daughter decreases Willpower Points.

"However, in contrast, *planning and prepping your food increases* your finite Willpower Points," he says. "Planning and prepping beautiful, healthy food to have available to eat is a nonnegotiable tenet in *Skinny School.* Many experts say that preparation is as much as *eighty-five percent of a person's success* in an endeavor."

That is a ridiculous statistic. I bet he is making that up.

"Let us begin our discussion about *planning and preparation.* Young Jackie, can you imagine an instructor having an expensive weekend seminar on investing and then showing up without a plan of what to teach? Or what about a successful college football coach coming to practice right before the bowl games without knowing what the team was going to work on that day? All Champions and winners have plans. They do not wing it. *Winging it means wrecking it.* Most dieters have no idea what they are going to eat each day, and as such, they have made no prior provisions. *That is not the way to succeed.* Learn from elite Champions. They plan. They prepare. *They do the work in advance to make sure things happen.* Tattoo that sentence on your brain. They do not just show up and see what rolls. Not knowing what you are going to eat each day and eating what is convenient is a recipe for disaster."

That is how I have lived my life for twenty-eight years.

"You understand this premise in other areas of your life. You plan for Christmas. You plan vacations. You plan the outline before you write legal briefs for Fortwright."

Actually, I am good at planning, but how does he know about Fortwright?

"The more you plan, *the less willpower you need to choose well.*"

This guy reminds me of the speeches of Martin Luther King, Jr. I am waiting for him to belt out, "I have a dream that one day, all women will be thin…"

"Mark it down—if you do not plan, *you will fail,*" he continues. "Your old downward pull of eating for pleasure and comfort will kick in. To override that beast, you must have a comprehensive plan in place."

Beast is a good description of my eating problem.

"Planning and preparation take work and effort, but Champions do not mind working for their goals. A Champion *Skinny School* student would never show up at dinnertime without a plan. That is ludicrous."

Eh…again…that is what I do every night.

"So tonight, we will address the beauty and majesty of planning and prepping as these two efforts determine a huge portion of your success," he says.

Didn't he say that ditching sugar and starches would determine a huge portion of my success?

"Genie, this sounds like it will take a lot of effort."

"Let us talk about *effort*," he says. "Huge goals require huge effort. But there is a lie in the American woman's mind that says her diet and food program should be easy and effortless. Where in life is accomplishing a big goal easy? Where? Do not begrudge the effort of working like a Champion. I will teach you to go the extra mile so you succeed. This one lie that eating right should not take much work undermines much of your success. The truth is that your degree of planning and prepping *will largely determine your success.*"

I doubt it. I mean, wouldn't Dr. Oz have talked about this if it were true?

"We will discuss three topics tonight," he says. "One, the importance of planning a Master Options List. Two, the necessity of constructing a Weekly Food Plan. And three, the imperative of planning and prepping a Daily Food Plan."

This is ridiculously excessive.

"Let us get started on topic one, the importance of planning a Master Options List, which is List Three in your Ruby Journal," he says. "This list is a list of all the food that you like and that is allowed. On the Master Options List, you list choices for breakfast, for lunch, and for dinner. This list will continue to grow and expand as you find new recipes that you love that are permissible. The idea here is that you have one place to collect your food choices, so you do not have to rethink a plan every time it is time to make a Weekly Food Plan."

A Weekly Food Plan? Should we not just start with one meal?

"The beauty of the Master Options List is that it will accumulate many choices for you and *choices are very important to humans.* Otherwise, rebellion often rears its ugly head."

I know all about rebellion.

"Human beings are programed for pleasure, so we are going to plan copious, beautiful food for you to keep around. After you have accumulated some recipes and food ideas on your Master Options List, you pick what recipes and foods you want to specifically have the next week and put them on your Weekly Food Plan. It is best to shop ahead for the entire week and have all needed ingredients in your house."

Won't my vegetables go bad in a week?

"Open your Ruby Journal to List Three, and entitle that page, 'Master Options List.' I have prepared a potential Master Options List of entrees for you, and I want you to diligently add to it as you discover other foods that you like that are healthy for you."

I open my Ruby Journal and begin to read:

List Three: Master Options List

Breakfast choices: Genie Vegetable Omelets; Genie Eggs Benedict with Hollandaise; scrambled eggs and bacon.[5]

Lunch options: Genie Spinach Salad with Bacon and Goat Cheese; Genie Deviled Eggs; Genie Deli Turkey Roll-Ups; Genie Chicken Vegetable Soup; Genie Grilled Chicken Salad with Pecans; Leftovers from dinner the night before are a favorite of other *Skinny School* students.

Dinner options: Literally unlimited! Genie Broiled Chicken Kebabs; Genie Dijon Butter Sauce; Genie Salmon; Genie Baked Orange Roughy; Genie Almond-Flour Fried Chicken; Genie Baked Flounder; Genie Rotisserie Chicken; Genie Steak with Genie Béarnaise sauce and so on.

Snack options: raw vegetables, 1 T. of peanut butter; ¼ cup of mixed nuts; apple; cup of vegetable soup.

---

5 All of the Genie recipes are located online at JulieNGordon.com/SkinnySchool.

"As you accumulate recipes, Young Jackie, you will list where the recipe is located, such as in what cookbook, where on the Internet, etcetera. Accumulating many delicious recipes will be extremely important to your success, so you do not give into boredom with eating the same thing."

But I don't like to plan my food. I like to wing it, because …planning is… well…work and restrictive.

"Remember, you have to have a magnificent plan that you can sustain, not a plan of deprivation. Giving up pizza, cheesecake, and homemade brownies is not such a big deal in light of having rich and satisfying foods prepared."

I think it is a big deal. Nothing short of a miracle is going to override my pattern of eating for pleasure and comfort. I hope he has some tricks up his sleeve.

"Scarcity breeds anxiety, so we will not focus on scarcity but on the galaxy of great food you can eat. I have developed a huge arsenal for you of delicious, healthy food choices."

Yeah, but not an arsenal of yummy carbs and sugars.

"The main purpose of food is nutrition," the Genie says. "The Creator made gorgeous, healthy food with stunning variety to delight you. You do not have to go outside His design to be satisfied. Giving up Trash Food such as simple starches and sweets will not be terribly difficult in the face of the beautiful recipes on your Master Options List."

I will believe it when I see it.

"Topic two is devising a Weekly Food Plan," he says. "Each week, I want you to take your Master Options List and make a Weekly Food Plan. Then you will need to go to the grocery store and get all the necessary ingredients for the entire week."

The entire week? Again—so overboard.

"Now we will discuss our third topic, Planning and Prepping the Day," he says. "Every day you will plan the food that you will eat. And in addition to planning it, you will prep it. This prepping step is crucial, but many ignore it. When the day presses in and it is time for lunch or dinner, even though a healthy meal is planned, few people will stop and do the needed chopping and prepping. You have to figure out when in your day you will prep the meals for the upcoming day's plan. Is it the night before? Is it early in the morning? You do not want to come home to an involved menu at six o'clock and know that you have to peel garlic, chop onions, and clean mushrooms. This is where *Champions separate from the average.* The work of prepping the night before or early in the morning is *the winner's edge.* Again, remember that this is a current Top Four Life Goal for you, and therefore you are willing to remove something else from your life so you can add *planning and prepping* your meals. Winners and Champions plan and prep!"

He acts like he thinks he is the president of the United States and he is doing the plan and prep work for something important, like a world-impacting discussion with other world leaders. This seems like overkill, honestly. I've read a thousand magazine articles on weight loss, and they all talk about calories and exercise, not his tomfoolery.

"If you fail to plan, you should plan to fail," he says. "And if you fail to prep, you should also plan to fail. Planning and prepping ahead add huge Willpower Points to your brain. There is a certain beauty and majesty about a beautiful plan and preparation of upcoming meals. It is like a fence around a schoolyard, giving the children freedom yet limits."

Ugh. I like freedom with no limits.

"When you come home after a long day, there must be some appropriate food planned and prepped, or *you will be in trouble.* That is all there is to it. You know that if you do not have good choices readily available when your Willpower Points are down, you are likely to fall in a ditch. But the dual skills of planning and prepping are new habits that you will have to master. You cannot wait and think about what you are going to eat when the moment arrives, *or you will most likely not make a good choice.* Successful *Skinny School* students have a written Master Options List, a Weekly Plan, and then a Daily Plan that is prepped. This makes all the difference in the world."

I might do that for a week, but seriously? He wants this to be a lifelong habit?

"Again, I cannot stress this truth enough," he says, "that opening the fridge door without a plan and prepped food when your Willpower Points are low is a surefire recipe for getting derailed. All your prior good intentions will disappear right there *if the prior work is not done.* Few humans can withstand moments of being tired and stressed and then have the willpower and energy to dig around and find appropriate food to eat. If you are not planned and prepared, you will fail, time and time again. *Success is found in planning and preparation.* Every success guru will tell you this. So repeatedly ask yourself, 'Where is my plan? Am I prepped for the day?'"

Having surfed the web about weight loss for years, I have never heard anyone babble on about planning and prepping like this dude. His advice is, well, doubtful, in my opinion.

"Of course, this is all a ridiculous oration on my part, Young Jackie, *unless you truly care about getting skinny.* Unless getting thin and healthy is in your current Top Four Life Goals, this is simply too much work. But if you do care and do not want to fall into the norm of eating Trash Food for comfort and entertainment, then you must be willing to go the extra mile and plan and prep."

Although it is true that being skinny is in my current Top Four Life Goals, I still want to find a way that is not so much work.

"The main point of today," he says, "is that Willpower Points are increased if food is planned and ready. It would be idiotic to not prethink and preplan if this is sincerely one of your Top Four Life Goals."

It seems like maybe he just called me an idiot.

"Now I am going to give you a power secret. Many *Skinny School* graduates attribute their success to this one secret."

Oh, yeah, sure.

"This power secret is called the Quart Bags. I insist that my *Skinny School* students make several Ziploc quart bags full of cleaned and prepared raw veggies every morning. This can be celery, mushrooms, cucumber slices, cherry tomatoes, romaine leaves, broccoli florets, etcetera. You can take veggies out of these bags to add to your meals, as well as use their contents for an emergency snack, such as when an anxiety moment arrives and you feel you must eat. This is a useful habit for life, as the fiber and nutrition in these veggies alone are worth the effort, not even counting how much fuller you will be if you eat raw vegetables every day."

Quart Bags? Of veggies? I want Quart Bags of cinnamon rolls.

"Surely situations come up when I cannot do all this planning and prepping," I say.

"We will thoroughly discuss all the nuances and challenges you will face as well as solutions to each dilemma, but one lesson at a time."

No one does all of this prepping. And I don't want to either.

"Just know that you will encounter much internal resistance to giving this huge amount of effort to planning and prepping your food, Young Jackie. But there is no other way. A woman will spend many hours helping a child finish his homework, a friend resolve a problem, or a nonprofit organization reach its goal. But she cannot justify spending two hours a week planning and shopping for one of her current Top Four Life Goals. She will often be reluctant to spend fifteen minutes in the morning to get her food prepped for the day. However, if you have diabetes, you take a shot. If your child has learning issues, you find ways to help him learn. *If you have compulsive overeating, you prep and plan.* Having healthy food available when it is time to eat is simply *nonnegotiable* if you want to overcome your eating problem. If you refuse to embrace this lesson, you will still be wrestling with your weight in five years."

What about thirteen years?

"To review one more time, Young Jackie, make a Master Options List, and then from this list, choose what you will eat for the next week's menu. Shop for those foods. Decide what you will eat for the next day, and prep the food needed. Many *Skinny School* students eat much the same thing during the day, but then they try to have a nice planned dinner to look forward to. I have left you a few Quart Bags with clean veggies in your fridge as well as my Genie Chicken Vegetable Soup for lunch tomorrow," he says and disappears.

Thinking about the two recent lessons that the Genie has now taught me, giving up sugar and refined carbs and planning/prepping like an OCD "Champion," I still feel like I have no idea what I am doing. The Genie did say that all the lessons work together, and around Lesson Seven, I should feel a "click" or a "flip" when I get it. Right now, I am still a million miles away from any "click" or "flip."

Realizing it is late, I decide to implement his ideas tomorrow. Grabbing some Breyer's chocolate-chip ice cream from my freezer, I take it to my bedroom. Immediate pleasure downloads into my brain. The fierce pleasure is intense and wonderful. After eating the whole bowl, I tiptoe back into the kitchen to get some more. I will start this whole *Skinny School* shebang tomorrow.

Lying down, I try to get comfortable, but my text message beep sounds. Huh…It is from an unknown number.

Starting on a program tomorrow will never give you results. Start now.

It is the Genie! This actually feels a little invasive of my privacy. I slowly savor the ice cream, but the text sort of spoils how good it tastes, since I feel that someone may be watching me.

There is my text message beep again. What does the Genie want to say now? Oh, dear. It is from Brandon.

What a great night. I felt something special was happening. Can't wait until Train.

Felt something special was happening? Maybe looking at my twenty-eight-year-old face all night made him feel young. I think looking at his forty-eight-year-old face all night made me feel old. Well, I do not know about successful, nice, good-mannered Gramps. He has got a long way to go. At least he likes *chubby* me.

I don't text back but turn off the light…again.

The nonnegotiables in *Skinny School* so far are:

1. I expect to work like a Champion to retrain my mind, since this is a current Top Four Life Goal.
2. Ditching sweets and starches is not optional if I want to overhaul my metabolism. I am to track my sugar/carb grams as well as my calories. I focus on all the beautiful, delicious food *I get to eat* instead of what I must not eat.
3. Planning and prepping are the secrets Champions use to conquer goals. I must daily make Quart Bags.

Lesson 4

Hunger IS Your Friend;

Tracking IS Your Friend

Monday, August 18   *Weight: 174*   *Pounds lost: 1*   *Still to lose: 44*

Driving up to the Michael E. Simpson Law Firm for my first day, I am nervous, just plain nervous. Really, it is stupid to be nervous when I think about it because if there is one thing I am good at, it is being a legal assistant. I guess the truth is I am nervous about whether the other employees will like me. I mean, Toothpick Eva has already let me know I'm not in her class. If I have to eat alone at lunch, then so be it.

Speaking of lunch, this whole *Skinny School* thing is taking a lot of time. I spent two hours yesterday planning, shopping, prepping, cooking, and packing. I made enough food last night so I would have leftovers for lunch today. Maybe once I get in a groove, it will not take as long, but for now, this assignment from the Genie is ultra time-consuming…and honestly annoying. But as Genie said yesterday, *"Champions work for their goals."* But this much? I started my Master Options List, wrote my Weekly Food Plan, shopped for it, and I actually have my Daily Food Plan written down and prepped. I got up early this morning and made a vegetable omelet. Also, I packed my lunch, a salad with tomatoes, cucumbers, and celery with hard-boiled eggs, grilled chicken, and two slices of bacon, along with some Caesar salad dressing. Also included were two snacks (a little bag of nuts and a piece of deli turkey meat rolled up with a slice of cheese on the inside). Shockingly, I have dinner prepped for when I get home, too. This is a little exhausting, but I must keep remembering, this is a current Top Four Life Goal, so I *should* spend time and energy on this. The Genie said the hardest part would be at first, learning the new thinking. He said, "I am not telling you it is going to be easy. *I am telling you it is going to be worth it.*"

Also I signed up for MyFitnessPal and have started tracking my foods. Fruit has so much sugar! And potatoes are full of carbs. This is a huge new learning curve.

To be honest, though, I already feel a tiny freedom. I mean, I have my food planned and prepped for the day. And when I eat every three hours (protein, veggies, and good fats), I do *not* have sugar cravings. Yesterday was the first day in a lonnng time that I did not cave in to sugar cravings. Drumroll, please! And I did lose the two pounds I gained plus one more, but that is probably just water.

Walking into the office early, I get to my desk and begin to rearrange a few things. Promptly at eight, Zach walks in. "Good morning, Jackie," he politely says. "Give me five minutes, and I will get you started on your day."

In exactly five minutes, Zach walks to my desk and begins to show me Amicus, the legal software. "This software program is what we used in Fortwright's office," I say. "I am familiar with it." He nods with approval.

Then Zach shows me his method to do intake on new clients. "I did intake on all of Fortwright's clients. I like that part of the job." He glances at me, again approvingly.

"Then you can get started on the demand packages," he says and gets up to return to his office. As he is getting up, he adds, "I will be in here working on a brief if you need me. Brief writing in probably the most unpleasant part of my job, but it has to be done."

"Do you want me to try to write your brief?" I ask.

Stopping, he turns around and stares at me. "Is that a joke? How would you know how to write a brief?"

I love this moment. Absolutely love it. Zach thinks it is impossible for a legal assistant to know how to write briefs. Why, law school has *courses* on brief writing and to think that an assistant could write a brief is ludicrous, I know. But Fortwright ordered a couple legal textbooks on brief writing and had me read them, and I have been writing briefs ever since. I have a natural proclivity for the law, anyhow. I just get law—what can I say? Fortwright used to say that the subject of law slid under the door and downloaded itself into my brain while I slept. Well, Zach, prepare to be stunned and amazed!

"I read two brief-writing textbooks, and then I wrote briefs for Fortwright all the time," I say casually but professionally. "Why don't you discuss the main tenets with me and give me a chance to write it for you?"

He stares at me with a stone face for a few seconds. Zach is not one to reveal his emotions, but I guess he is probably thinking he made a mistake hiring a deluded assistant like me...one who thinks she can write legal briefs.

"All right, come into my office, and we will give this a try," he says. I immediately like this about him, the fact that he is not closed-minded to something seemingly outrageous.

Eva walks in at that minute, and just the sight of her makes my heart drop. She is sporting a purple knit dress that clings tightly to her body, with four-inch black stilettos. Her earrings are black and purple, a perfect addition to make her outfit sparkle. Here I am in my frumpy brown pants and cream tunic with this paisley scarf. In her presence, I feel like a big brown bear that has escaped from the zoo.

Mumbling a quick "Hey" to me without a smile, she walks into Zach's office. In a whisper (which I can hear), she says, "Today is our foursome's lunch, Zach. Can you meet at Rafferty's at noon?"

He does not lower his voice. "Not today, sorry. This brief is weighing on me."

Sighing, she exits his office, kind of like a dog with its tail between its legs. The little puppy did not get the bone she wanted.

Trying to not let the discouragement of her tiny body overwhelm me, I gather myself and enter Zach's office. He goes over the points, telling me about the case law, giving me direction, and then I go back to my desk. Concentrating, I become focused in a crazy way. Writing is one place where I can fire on all cylinders.

Two hours later, I e-mail Zach my first draft. Walking to the door of his office, I lightly say, "Zach, I e-mailed you the first few pages of the brief. Will you read it, please? I want to be sure I am headed in the direction you wanted."

Returning to my desk, I wait. I hate to admit this, but I am pretty excited about what is getting ready to happen.

Predictably, it happens. Five minutes later, Zach walks to my desk and just stares. "I have never heard of a legal assistant who can write briefs. This is excellent writing, Jackie. Excellent. I am stunned, to be honest."

That is what I was waiting on. I might be fat, but I have got a good brain.

"This is my lucky day," he says, shaking his head. "Gallons of my stress have been removed. I am shocked you can write like this."

Although I may not be able to rock wearing purple knit dresses, I can rock writing legal briefs. And now Zach knows it.

We talk for another ten minutes about a few changes and more case law.

While we are talking, a delivery man appears at my doorway with two dozen yellow roses in his arms. "These are for Jackie Holbrook," he says.

Embarrassed, I immediately know whom they are from. Receiving the bouquet, I quickly read the card: THINKING OF YOU AND SENDING GOOD WISHES ON YOUR FIRST DAY. BRANDON.

Gulp. I hate this. Trying to play it low-key on my first day, I instead get this ridiculous, ostentatious bouquet of yellow roses. Zach goes back into his office as if he has not noticed. All-business Zach. Of course.

Eva wanders in again. "Who are the flowers from?" she pries.

"Just a friend," I say, as if I am going to tell *her* anything.

Entering Zach's office again, she asks, "Zach, can I bring you some take-out from Rafferty's?" She is like a persistent mosquito.

Eva follows Zach to my desk, where he hands me some more minor corrections on the brief. "No thanks, Eva." He returns to his desk, and there she is, still standing in my office.

"If you ever go to Rafferty's, Jackie, you should order their potato-cheese soup. It is one of their signature dishes," she says, as she begins to leave.

Not really thinking about her comment, I reply, "Oh, is that what you order when you go?"

"Oh, heavens, no," she squeals. "That soup has *way* too many calories in it for me. I just thought *you* might like it." And she exits.

Moments like this have the power to make me want to fall down into a deep well and never crawl out again. What a dig. She might as well have said, "You obviously do not care about what you eat, so here is a tip for some food for a fattie." Finding a way to get along with Eva is going to be the rough part of this job. Her comment was mean, and I expect more are forthcoming.

All the rest of the day, I plow and plod and think and write. At five o'clock, Zach walks to my desk. "I cannot tell you how much I appreciate this excellent work, Jackie. Hiring you was one of the smartest things I have done in a long time," he says with the slightest of grins on his face. Looking at his smooth, dark skin and his shiny gray-green eyes, I sort of tremble.

Tongue-tied, I say, "Thank you. I like being here." I smile my prettiest smile. My very, very prettiest one. He is not afraid to make eye contact. At least we are going to be good professional friends. He respects me, and I… well, I think he is one beautiful specimen of a male human being.

As I gather my purse to leave, Eva walks in again and begins telling Zach a story about big brown bears tap dancing, and she begins to "tap dance" to explain one part. Obviously, it is a ploy to make him notice her legs. Feeling a little sick, I, the big brown bear, exit for the day.

"Oh, Jackie," Eva calls after me. "Daddy—I mean, Attorney Simpson—told me to tell everyone that we are having the annual Employee Appreciation Dinner next Friday night, the 29th, at the Capitol Grille restaurant. Are you free? You can bring a date. Bring the guy who sent you the flowers, so we can all meet him."

Horrors. I am not bringing Gramps anywhere. "I can come, but I will be alone. That was just a friend who sent the flowers," I say. It was an aged friend whose memory is probably on the decline and who will not even remember sending them. There I go again, being hard on Brandon. Actually, he is decently bright and certainly treats me well. *What is my problem?* The thought that guys like Zach Boltz are my problem enters my brain, but I quickly dismiss that. Fat girls do not get guys like Zach Boltz. And besides, he already has a girlfriend, charming Rachel, as if I could ever compete with her. The Genie and his promises about changing my metabolism—and then my body dropping eons of weight—enter my mind, giving me the tiniest glimpse of hope in someday conquering my volcano-sized problem and finding my own Prince Charming.

Driving home, I dissect the mixed feelings about my first day. Yes, I am pleased that Zach likes my work. But putting up with Eva is going to be a stretch. The traffic is bad, and I am very tired and emotionally depleted. It is kind of sad that I do not get bread and dessert anymore. I love chocolate cake, and sandwiches on thick, sourdough bread, and cupcakes, and bakery chocolate-chip cookies...

Glancing at my passenger seat, I am startled as there is the Genie! He is in his usual high-energy state, which is quite a contrast to how depleted I feel.

"I thought I would take advantage of this bad traffic, and we would have Lesson Four, Hunger is Your Friend."

Is driving and having a Genie in your front seat as dangerous as driving and texting?

"Humans have been given a mechanism by the Creator that tells them when to eat," he says as he jumps right into the topic. "It is called *hunger*."

I thought the best way to eat was on a three-hour schedule, like all the TV shows and magazines say to do.

"Humans also have a mechanism that tells them when to *stop* eating. It is the point at which *they are no longer hungry*—not when they are, as is commonly thought, *full*."

Of course everyone eats until they are full. This is rubbish.

"First, wait until you are truly physically hungry to eat," he says. "Secondly, eat beautiful, nutritious proteins, fats, and vegetables, not sweets or starches. And thirdly, stop when you are *no longer hungry,* not when you are full. You will lose weight, regain much emotional stability, and acquire a new sense of freedom."

Poppycock and nonsense. He is making all this up.

"*Physical* hunger must be distinguished from *emotional* hunger," he says, "which is when you want to eat to either soothe or entertain yourself. You probably have not been physically hungry in a long time."

I am not even sure I remember what physical hunger feels like.

"A scale exists," he says, "between one and ten that will help you determine when to eat and when to stop. Ten is so stuffed that you feel sick. Nine is very similar. Eight is very, very full. Seven is full. Six is a little bit full. Five is the point at which you still cannot feel the food in your stomach, but you are no longer hungry. *It is at a five that you stop eating.* Four is not hungry, but you definitely could eat. Three is where you feel the first sensation of true physical hunger and you are allowed to eat. Two is very hungry, and at this point, food is primarily all you are thinking about. If you wait until you are a one, that is getting into the ravenous zone, and that is too long to wait."

How am I supposed to remember his little half-baked chart?

"*Eat when you become a three, a two-point-five, or a two. Then eat nutritious, appetizing, and savory food until you are at a five. Then do not eat again until you are at a three or lower.*"

First, he says no sugar. Then he says plan and prep like a Champion. Now his cockamamie advice is to wait until I am hungry to eat. Surely I am not to believe this hooey. Where is my twelve-hundred-calorie diet and a cardio workout like all the experts of the world decree?

"Young Jackie, you will enjoy food more than you ever have before if you wait until you are hungry to eat. Hunger is the best sauce in the world. Even simple foods taste *exquisite* when you are truly hungry."

This kooky guy is wearing me out with his screwball advice.

"You will discover that *it does not take much food* to get you from a three to a five," he says. "You will need to slow down and savor each bite. Eating slowly is very important because you are looking for that point *before* you are full, the point at which you are *no longer hungry.* It takes around twenty minutes for the food in your stomach to tell your brain that you have had enough. This is a big learning curve for you, Young Jackie."

This is the flakiest diet information I have ever heard.

"Learning how to eat delicious, nutrient-dense food when you are hungry and to stop before you can feel the food in your stomach is the most freeing, slenderizing, and actually healthy way to eat in the world. This is how a skinny, healthy mind-set thinks," he says.

This is how a UFO mind-set thinks.

"Not only does hunger make food taste exceptional," he says, "but slowing down and actually paying attention to *taste* your food—instead of inhaling it—will doubly increase your enjoyment of it."

I have enjoyed my Trash Food plenty, thank you; it is just the aftereffects that I do not enjoy.

"You will discover," the Genie says, "that you are tempted to eat numerous times during the day *besides* when you are physically hungry. The Creator made the hunger mechanism so you would eat when it goes off. You are not to eat otherwise."

Oh, no. One of those outlandish statements again. I wish he would quit making those absurd statements.

"Saying goodbye to feeling full is difficult, I admit, because, being full with large quantities of food does quickly dial down your emotions," he says.

That's the first true thing he has said in a long time! And what is going to replace that, may I ask?

"How deceiving, though, is that temporary escape from your problems," he says. "The truth is that eating large amounts of food does not get you what you *truly* want most: thinness! You are trading a temporary escape from your problems for a lifetime of chubbiness! Instead, you must find legitimate ways to deal with your emotions instead of *eating them away.*"

Alcohol is not a healthy solution. Drugs are out. Overspending got me in trouble a few years ago. What else is there besides unhealthy addictions?

"Tell me what to do when I feel the world caving in," I throw out. I need another strategy to survive the emotional traumas of life since I will no longer have my buddy, food.

"We will discuss several ideas in upcoming lessons, but for now, if you cannot dial down an emotional tsunami *and feel you must eat,* then eat out of your Quart Bags. Another great thing to do when you are not physically hungry but emotionally hungry is to drink herbal teas. The fabulous flavors range from vanilla chocolate to red raspberry. These herbal teas are actually healthy and can soothe ruffled emotions. Add a little non-GMO stevia, a brand like Sweet Leaf, and you have a delicious, soothing drink. Also, sometimes a hot vegetable soup broth will soothe you if you need a little warmth and stomach filler. Many *Skinny School* graduates sip herbal teas and soup broths during the day, as well as crunch on some of the veggies from their Quart Bags, waiting on hunger."

At least there is something I can put in my mouth when I feel I might jump off a cliff. But thinking about the Genie's *Skinny School* and his advice, I wonder if I can do all of this. Maybe this whole idea that I could ever be thin is ludicrous. Maybe I am destined to be a chub. His so-called secrets and lessons are hard and difficult to get my mind around.

"When the idea to eat arises, just ask yourself, *Am I truly physically hungry?*" he says. "That is all you have to do. And if you truly are a three or lower, then eat what you have planned on your Daily Food Plan."

I have been eating when I wanted for twenty-eight years, and now he wants me wait until I am physically hungry to eat. Not gonna be easy.

"If you are going to exercise and your stomach hurts when it is empty," he says, "eat a teaspoon of natural peanut butter. You do not have to be perfect on this program. Just get the mind-set that when you can, you wait on hunger, you wait on hunger, you wait. It is the number one most important secret of weight loss, to wait on hunger. Wait, wait, wait. Wait until you are hungry."

First he said ditching sweets and starches was the most important secret of weight loss. Then he said planning and prepping was the most important principle. Now he says to wait on hunger. He should make up his mind.

"In the musical *Mary Poppins*, she quotes an old English proverb that says, 'Enough is as good as a feast.' Think about what that means. If you have tasted the food and are no longer hungry, then moderation and 'enough' is as good as a feast. Stop before you are full."

But I like getting full.

"If you are eating out, immediately divide your plate into halves," he says. "You can box up half of your dinner and use it for another meal. Restaurants have a habit of serving too much food. You are in charge of how much you eat, not the person who serves your food."

Large portions make me happy. Well, at least while I am eating them.

"Let's review Lessons One through Four, Young Jackie. Lesson One was to determine your current Top Four Life Goals, so you would grasp how important being thin is to you, as well as helping you realize that of course you are willing to do a great deal of work to attain one of these goals. Lesson Two was to ditch sweets and starches and instead to eat mouthwatering, nutrient-dense food such as proteins, good fats, and vegetables. Lesson Three was to construct a Master Options List, a Weekly Food Plan, and then to devise a Daily Food Plan, which is a list of food planned and prepped for your day. Today's lesson, Lesson Four, is to wait until you are truly physically hungry and to stop before you are full."

Work. Work. Work.

"Young Jackie, you now eat in response to a desire to self-soothe, to medicate some unpleasant feelings, or to entertain or stimulate yourself. Instead, you must learn to eat in response to physical hunger. Finding other outlets or activities for self-soothing and entertaining yourself is another topic, which we will discuss in detail in Lesson Seven, Finding Substitutes for Self-Soothing and Entertainment."

Lesson Seven? I need that information now.

"When you do realize that you are truly physically hungry, do not dive into the food," he says. "Become incredibly conscious and intentional about eating. Decide to eat *gently*. Of course, you will have wholesome food available from your Daily Food Plan, as you have planned and prepped your food. So when real hunger strikes, it is important to slow down the tiger in you that wants to rip the food apart with your bare teeth. Self-control and mindfulness are needed, paying attention to when the 'five' moment arrives, in which you are no longer hungry."

Like right now—I am not physically hungry, but eating is what I want to do. How will I ever change this pattern?

"What you will notice, Young Jackie, is that the first bites of food eaten when you are truly, physically hungry, are sensational. Just outrageously delicious. But you will also notice that enjoyment diminishes after each bite. This is why it is imperative that you eat slowly and consciously, paying attention to your food."

Eating at the speed of light, I often don't even taste my food.

"Wise women know that the food they eat and the amount they eat are about so much more than the momentary taste," he says. "Choosing not to eat until you are physically hungry and then stopping before you are full is really a choice about what kind of body you will live in, to experience your one and only precious life."

My one and only precious life has so far been lived in a German tank.

"This may be the hardest tenet in *Skinny School* to adopt," he says. "Humans do not want to stop when they are enjoying something, but they can learn to do so. Self-control is a fabulous virtue, getting you what you really want."

"Won't there be times when I can't wait until I am hungry to eat?" I ask. "For example, when I am on a trip with other people, and they are getting ready to eat and I'm not truly hungry. What do you do then?" Now he will understand what a ridiculous program this is and how inconvenient.

"Of course those situations will happen," he says, "and I will discuss all of that strategy in upcoming lessons. But for now, *do the best you can* in these difficult situations until I give you exact strategies in how to handle them."

Holding in my objections no longer, I blurt out, "Genie, this is all so much work!" Okay, there, I said it.

He pauses and looks intently at me before speaking. "Why would you expect something as valuable as being thin to be easy? Why do you expect to gain something without effort? It is as though you have a brain block about this. In every other area of your life, you realize that it is a sowing and reaping world, Young Jackie. But with your food, you are still thinking like a child, wanting something without paying the price. Women will go to the ends of the earth for their children, friends, and employers. But they are reluctant to take two hours a week to plan and shop, and they are reluctant to take fifteen minutes in the morning to plan for the day, prep the ingredients, pack their lunches, make their Quart Bags, and read their Ruby Journals for daily motivation. Never do I claim that that *Skinny School* is easy; I claim that if you work the program, you can change how you think about food and be thin for the rest of your life."

The feeling that overtakes me as he says this is sharp and a little gut wrenching. I feel exposed. It is like I have had my photo taken without makeup on. Or like my dirty bra strap is showing. The Genie has hit the proverbial nail on the head, and that nail is my laziness, my wanting things to be easy without paying the price. Intellectually, I know better. I mean, I know you can't learn French without effort. But somewhere in my brain, there is this thought that weight loss should come easily. It is as though eating what and when I want should be included in the Bill of Rights: "Life, liberty, the pursuit of happiness, and to eat what and when I want." Genie is blowing that false thinking up. I have not had the right thinking, and he is trying to train my brain to have it. I do want thinness. I do. So now I have to ask myself, am I willing to pay this price of relearning how to think about food so that I can, once and for all, be done with this garbage of being a fattie?

The answer I hear myself say is a loud yes, yes, and yes. I will do this. I was thinking what a hassle this was, but actually, it is a life gift. Yes, this is a life gift…to train my brain how to think right so I can be thin forever. My lower self's desire for life to be an easy and paved highway will never go away. I must accept that to be thin, I am going to have to do battle. These sermons of the Genie are redundant but necessary.

"The media is continually exhorting people to watch portion size," he says. "If you will monitor your fullness carefully, you will see that portion size shrinks exponentially. It takes very little food to satisfy hunger. Your previous large portions were not to satisfy your hunger; they were attempts to satisfy your need for soothing and stimulation. I will say this a hundred times in *Skinny School*: *you must find substitutes for your legitimate needs of soothing and stimulation besides food.* We will discuss this more thoroughly in Lesson Seven."

He keeps postponing discussing the important stuff, if you ask me.

"We have to discuss one more topic today that is actually somewhat of a review," the Genie says.

Surely that was enough for one day.

"I have made List Four in your Ruby Journal and entitled it 'Tracking Your Hunger.'"[6].

"When you get home," he continues, "you can look at it. It is just a chart where you *track your hunger*. I know there is a lot of tedious work in *Skinny School* right now, but these behaviors are imperative for a short time, so you can uncover how you deceive yourself. Tracking is a tool that bursts through your avoidance strategies and makes you face all the deceptive ploys you do to yourself. Tracking is your friend because it keeps you from going 'unconscious' and reverting back to your prior habits. I will tell you this with certainty: your lower self, which we will discuss in the next lesson, will resist tracking. Tracking makes you accountable to yourself, and there is a part of you that does not want to be accountable to anyone, even yourself."

True. Very true.

"You will notice on your Tracking Sheet that you are going to pay attention to your hunger. Once again I remind you this is a current Top Four Life Goal, and you are trying to get free from the ball and chain of chubbiness for life, so it is definitely worth the work. I am asking you to track your food intake as well as your hunger during *Skinny School* so you can see the traps you fall into. Then you will be able to make decisions that are more in line with your current Top Four Life Goals. Even though you will resist tracking your hunger and your food intake, *you must find a way to do this*, as this exercise will give you invaluable feedback. How do you expect to change habits if you will not face what you are doing now?"

Uh, well, I…hmm. I do not know.

"Human beings are such an oddity," he says. "You have self-destructive behaviors, and then, because it is uncomfortable to face this truth, you try to avoid thinking about your damaging behaviors."

I have always known that other people have blind spots, but I guess I thought I was too smart to do that. Obviously not.

---

6 You can download a free sample Tracking Sheet at JulieNGordon.com/SkinnySchool

"This is a large amount of new information, so I hope you will review it a few times. Remember, Young Jackie, when you lose your way, return to this Miraculous Threesome: Ditch (sweets and starches), Plan, and Wait. These three concepts are the foundation of *Skinny School*. When you feel discouraged or make a bad choice, immediately return to the Miraculous Threesome to get back on the path. I left a recipe of Genie Salmon in your fridge. I will return soon," and he departs.

Arriving at my apartment, I feel almost dazed with all my new material to process. Entering the kitchen, I cut up celery sticks, clean cherry tomatoes, slice cucumber slices, as well as clean some mushrooms. I gulp them all down like I am in a contest to see how fast I can finish. I am crazy, I know. I was supposed to wait until I was hungry to eat, but the Genie said I can eat out of my Quart Bags if I am in an emotional frenzy, and I guess I am in one.

There is a ravenous animal inside of me that, at this point, knows no other way to self-soothe except to eat. My emotional discomfort has been quelled by eating large amounts for many years. At least the large amounts of raw vegetables that I just ate are friendly to my new plan. The insanity edge is now off. I hope to learn how to dial down my internal ravenous animal eventually, but at least today I slowed the animal and calmed him with the Quart Bags. I do see the merit of the Quart Bags; I just do not quite know if I am disciplined enough to plan and prep like the Genie suggested. And now I am supposed to wait to eat until I am at a three or below? Holy smokes, this feels like a noisy gong clanging in my brain. I don't want to do all this, but honestly, there is not another way. I have looked for one for thirteen years, and there is not one.

My cell is ringing, and it's Beth. She is calling as she drives to a wine-tasting event to meet her husband, Richard. When I met Beth, she did not drink alcohol, but since Richard is a food and wine gourmet, she frequently now has a glass or two of wine. Alcohol is one of those subjects that usually separates "those who do" from "those who do not," but Beth and I have managed to overlook each other's preference. Beth wants to hear all about the first day.

"How did you do with Eva today?" is her question. Of course, any bona fide best friend would ask that.

"It was good except one moment," I say, as I tell her about the potato-cheese soup episode.

"Low," she oozes, "very low."

Even though I know that I will eventually have to find the energy to "return good for evil" in my relationship with Eva, it is soothing to have a friend who understands the pain of being treated rudely.

"Not going to be easy if she keeps that up," I add, hoping to get a little more pity.

"You will rise to the occasion and respond well eventually," my wise friend says. "No one does well with a surprise pie in their face."

Beth is a great friend on many levels, but entering into my trials is at the top of her virtues.

Brandon is beeping in, but I let it go to voice mail. Earlier I texted him a quick, **Thank you for the beautiful roses.** What does Gramps want now? To borrow a cane? I get a little uneasy thinking about Gramps. I wonder if he will grow on me. The flowers were overboard, but old guys do not understand you need to play it cool. Maybe they think they might die soon, so there is no time to waste.

Listening to Gramps's voice mail, in which he rambles a lot about nothing, I know that my feelings for him are definitely going to need a boost if this is going to work.

The thought that I would like to eat surfaces, but I quickly realize I am not physically hungry but only wanting to soothe myself. Opening my Quart Bags, I grab a handful of celery and glance at my Daily Food Plan to see what is written down for dinner. I have planned to eat a little leftover Genie Chicken Vegetable Soup from yesterday, a large salad, some cauliflower with a little cheese, and finish with a few nuts.

Instead of eating like I normally would, I make some herbal tea to take with me as I head for the mall. What I wore to Fortwright's office did not matter because whatever I wore was better than his wrinkly suits and the faded wingback chairs. But now, the ante has been upped. Now I am around Calvin Klein Eva, with all her fashionable purring. Time to step up my fashion game.

Trying on a few pairs of slacks, I get discouraged. It is like a hippopotamus trying to put on a toddler outfit. How I hate being chubby and shopping for clothes!

Hearing my text message, I take it out of my purse. Probably Brandon bugging me again. Oh, my goodness. It is from Zach!

I would like you to go with me in the morning to take some pictures of an accident scene. I can show you how I like them done, so you can do them by yourself in the future. We can use the time in the car to talk more about the brief.

I have taken enough photos of accident scenes that I could take them while simultaneously painting my nails and standing on my head. But I will not brag about that to Zach. I will let him teach me. Heavens! In the car, alone with Zach? The thought both horrifies me and excites me, all at once. If only I could lose forty pounds by morning!

What is that feeling I am experiencing? Why, it is hunger! I am actually feeling hunger! I will go home and eat my dinner. Wow, this is new. Hunger. I have not felt this sensation in a while. I cannot wait to eat! Yippee!

The nonnegotiables in *Skinny School* so far are:

1. I expect to work like a Champion to retrain my mind since this is a current Top Four Life Goal.
2. Ditching sweets and starches is not optional if I want to overhaul my metabolism. I am to track my sugar/carb grams as well as my calories. I focus on all the beautiful, delicious food *I get to eat* instead of what I must not eat.
3. Planning and prepping are the secrets Champions use to conquer goals. I must daily make Quart Bags.
4. Hunger is my friend, and waiting until I am truly hungry to eat and quitting before I am full are nonnegotiable. Tracking my hunger is imperative and will expose how I deceive myself with wanting to eat for self-soothing and entertainment.

Lesson 5

Understanding the Tricks of Your Demanding Child Personality

Friday, August 22   *Weight: 172*   *Pounds lost: 3*   *Still to lose: 42*

Zach and I were supposed to take pictures of an accident scene last Tuesday, but it poured down rain. We put off the photo session until today because he was busy all week preparing for a trial—which ended up being postponed. Zach is a machine as far as grinding out the work, but I can grind it out, too. And Zach likes that about me. And I like that he likes it.

My weight loss has me a little pumped. I have lost five pounds since last Saturday (well, counting the two I had just gained). I have been working it, though, like a true Champion. I wait until I am truly physically hungry, and then I eat chicken, broccoli with cheese sauce, salads galore, steak, flounder, eggs, cut-up veggies, nuts, or a tiny bit of quiche. This definitely has *not* been deprivation. *It is just so much work to get my food ready.*

However, I am somewhat willing to do this work and learn new habits because I am sick of being fat. How ridiculous of me *to want the prize without paying the price*, but that is what I have been doing for thirteen years. I admit, the time I spend planning, shopping, prepping, and cooking is outrageous, but I keep in mind the word *Champion*. I remember how much energy elite Champions put into their goals. Hopefully, one day, this will be a way of life and will not require this kind of focus.

The work of planning and prepping is bad enough, but what is really hard about *Skinny School* is waiting to eat until I am physically hungry. When I want to eat, I ask myself if I am physically hungry, and the answer is usually no. However, some emotion is aroused in me that is uncomfortable, and I realize I want to use food *to change the way I feel*. This one principle in *Skinny School* will be as difficult to master as the others combined. Thank goodness I have my Quart Bags when I feel I *must* eat.

Zach asks if I can be ready at 10:00 a.m. We leave, and he begins discussing another brief that is due in three weeks. I take notes as he talks. At the accident scene, Zach begins to "train me" by telling me about getting this view and that angle. I have to muzzle my mouth not to give *him* a few pointers on how to take the pictures of accident scenes.

"I am hungry," he says. "Let's stop at the Midtown Café for lunch."

My brain begins to buzz. What will I eat there? Will they have food on my plan? My prepped lunch is at the office, and I was not ready to eat out, although I am truly hungry.

My silence throws him. "What's wrong?" he asks. "Do you already have lunch plans?"

"Oh, no," I say, slowly, debating what to tell him. Why put up a front? It is easy to see I need to lose weight so I decide to be honest. "I'm on a weight loss program where I count my carb and sugar grams, so I was just thinking if the Midtown Café would have food I could eat. But of course, they will have a salad with grilled salmon or chicken, so let's stop."

He glances at me to try to read if I am being sincere or just accommodating. My expression must have convinced him I want to stop, because he just nods his head and drives toward the restaurant. Zach does not waste time or energy on excess words.

His tan, strong hands firmly hold the steering wheel, and his dark hair hangs a little bit over his ears. His pressed slacks and Johnson Murphy tassel loafers look regal. Honestly, it is all a little too much to take in.

Glancing down at my excess forty pounds, a feeling of discouragement sweeps over me. Here I am, with one of the most attractive men that I have ever been around, and I am a chunk who is far from his league. Pulling my mind away from that thought, I tell myself that I am now on a good program and command myself to not let discouragement descend.

Once we are seated, Zach and I order, and then I excuse myself to go to the ladies' room, where I powder my nose and reapply lipstick. I may as well look as good as I can from the neck up.

"What was it like working for Fortwright?" Zach asks when I return. Even in this short time of knowing Zach, I realize he is not looking for gossip; he is simply trying to have a nice conversation.

I fall into a lavish description of the difference of the faded plaid wingback chairs versus the highbrow leather of our current office. Then I lapse into stories about when I started there years ago. For example, I tell Zach how the fish were dead for two weeks in the aquarium before anyone fished them out. And I tell him how the secretary would not write down appointments, and then Fortwright would close the office at three o'clock, thinking he was giving the employees a treat, but thereby leaving clients knocking at a locked door.

Zach is not just grinning; he is laughing. He thinks I'm funny.

On and on I blabber. Gosh, I must really work on talking too much.

"Where did you get this understanding of law?" he asks before I can ask him a question. He is interested in what I say, so again I start a monologue, telling him about how Fortwright liked me to learn everything in the office. (I am careful how I say this, trying to protect Fortwright's problem.) Then I tell Zach how I am now studying for the LSAT to go to law school myself. Oops. There I go again, rambling on about myself.

But Zach's face says he is not annoyed in the least. In fact, he seems to enjoy me.

"There is a website that I used to study for the LSAT," he says. "I will send you the link. You would be a great lawyer, Jackie."

I feel embarrassed talking about myself so much, but his sentence about what a great lawyer I would be elevates my mood several notches. What a compliment, coming from Zach. His dark, gray-green eyes are not afraid to be friendly and meet mine. He is interested in what I say, and he thinks I am funny. Again I am aware that we are going to be friends, at least in a professional sense.

"How did you decide to go to law school?" I ask, finally getting the conversation off me. Zach begins a long story about teaching tennis for three years after college, wrestling with the decision, and navigating his parents' subsequent involvement in his decision. We chat like friends, not like boss and employee. He seems like he is not in a hurry. Honestly, I am surprised that Business Zach is so personable. I like the way he thinks before he talks, that he talks in organized paragraphs—and yet he has no apparent shield over his heart, just letting what is down in the well come up in the bucket.

The bill comes and I reach for my purse.

"No Jackie, you don't pay when we are out on business," he says, matter-of-factly.

If only we could be out when it *was not* business, I dream, knowing that will never happen.

The thought then comes to my mind that I cannot ever remember enjoying anyone's company more in my life. The word *Rachel* was never even mentioned. I mean, that is his personal life; why would we talk about his girlfriend? We are business associates. Anyhow, I am sure they will be engaged any minute now. Is that not what people do when they have dated two years and they are twenty-eight and thirty years old?

Thinking of weddings, Attorney Simpson's son—Eva's brother—is getting married in three weeks, and the entire office is invited, including me. I think about how much weight I can lose before that event. And then I remember the Employee Appreciation Dinner is coming up this Friday, and I will get to see ravishing Rachel again. That thought is a definite downer.

Back in the car, Zach takes a call from a potential new client, and I check my e-mail on my phone. Brandon has forwarded me an article on Train. The poor guy is trying so hard. Maybe I should consider taking Jessica's advice and give him a chance.

All-business Zach and I return to our respective desks, grinding out the afternoon's work.

Quitting time comes, and Eva, as usual, enters Zach's office. This time it is a tightrope story, and she illustrates the story by demonstrating how she is balancing on a tightrope, again drawing attention to her award-winning legs. "Are you bringing Rachel to the dinner Friday night?" she squeaks.

"Rachel is going to be out of town," he says.

You could actually hear the delight in Eva's voice. "Really?" she says, just as if he had said, "I have a five hundred dollar gift certificate for you from Neiman Marcus."

I criticize Eva in my mind for being excited about him not bringing Rachel. But—the truth is, *I feel exactly the same way.* Realizing how much I enjoy and crave Zach's company, I feel stupid, as if there could ever be any more relationship than mere business associates.

As I head home in the rush-hour traffic, the Genie appears in my passenger seat. Maybe I should be getting used to this, but I'm not.

"Today's lesson is often the one that begins to flip the switch," he begins. "This lesson allows women to see that winning the weight battle is all in your thoughts. I recommend listening very carefully to today's lesson. *You will miss the heart of* Skinny School *if you miss today's lesson.*"

He acts like he thinks he is the pope.

"Humans have two natures, Young Jackie," he says. "They have a lower nature, which we will call the Demanding Child. This nature always presses for immediate gratification. It is completely concerned with whatever feels easy and good *now*. In contrast, humans have a higher nature, which I will call the Sane Adult. This nature is concerned about reaching important goals. The battle between your two natures makes you feel a little crazy at times."

A little crazy? How about stark-raving mad?

"Although your Sane Adult and your Demanding Child both sound like you because their voices sound the same, *they are from two different parts of your brain.* As time goes by, you will get more adept at identifying who is speaking in your brain, either your Sane Adult or your Demanding Child."

What hooligan stuff is he now trying to say?

"One huge trick that your Demanding Child uses to get you to eat when you are not hungry," he says, "is that she persuades you to soothe yourself from your emotional distress with food. Your Demanding Child will list all your problems, tell you how burdensome they are, and thus insist that you medicate your uncomfortable feelings by eating them down. Your Demanding Child will remind you that you just wasted six months on a loser boyfriend, that you have to deal with an unpleasant roommate, and that you no longer have a mother to comfort you. *Self-pity is a very effective tool Demanding Child uses to get you to eat when you are not physically hungry."*

He did not even mention Eva in that list of woes. Now I have to put up with her daily meanness and all those ridiculous outfits.

The Genie continues, "'Trash Food,' your Demanding Child whispers, 'will make you feel better.' And guess what, Young Jackie? She is right! Trash Food will make you feel better...for about one or two minutes, the time spent while actually eating the food. But this whole situation is insane! *She convinces you to enjoy two minutes of pleasure or comfort at the expense of one of your current Top Four Life Goals!* That is insanity thinking!"

Eh, that is how I think all the time.

"Take each of Demanding Child's tricks and bring it to light," he says. "There are not two thousand tricks, but around twenty," he says. "In your Ruby Journal, make a new list. Entitle it, 'List Five: Repeated Schemes My Demanding Child Uses.' Write down the schemes of Demanding Child and then counteract those tricks by writing down the truth of your Sane Adult's thinking. This will enable you to see Demanding Child's insanity and instead choose what is best for you long-term."

Tricks? Schemes? What is this nonsense?

"Mentally fight your Demanding Child each moment she appears," he says. "Yes, initially, during the two to three minutes that everyone else is eating dessert, you will experience some discomfort. But Champions withstand short-term discomfort *all the time* for the prize. Your Sane Adult is *more than willing* to give up a temporary food sensation for the grand prize of skinniness."

Withstanding discomfort is not in my strength set.

"This is where Champions separate from others," he says. "Your Sane Adult truly wants thinness, so pledge to redouble your efforts. Clear more of your schedule to make the time to plan, shop, and prep. Read your Ruby Journal two or three times a day to strengthen your resolve and motivation.

That is what humans do for their Top Four Life Goals. Get rid of the unnecessary activities in your life, so you can create margins to accomplish this goal. Do not let any obstacle take you down. Do not let your whiney Demanding Child throw any of her excuses at you."

I am a paralegal, not LeBron James.

"Demanding Child will sulk and bemoan how deprived she feels that she ate celery while everyone else was eating cupcakes," he says. "That is not what your Sane Adult thinks. Your Sane Adult says, 'Bravo for doing what you need to do to go after what you really want: thinness!' Your Sane Adult wants you to have a will of steel that refuses to give in to some short-lived taste experience."

My will is more like Jell-O.

"Sane Adult is *not* looking at the price she has to pay or the sacrifice; she is looking at accomplishing the goal, *the beautiful, luxurious goal of skinniness.* Champion thinkers have long ago left whining and complaining in the dust. They know that *of course* there is a price to pay. Of course, there is a sacrifice. And they are delighted to pay it because in exchange, they get a treasure chest of prizes, which in your case, is thinness."

I want a treasure chest *without* paying any price.

"Demanding Child will repeatedly tell you how unfair it is that you have to struggle with many disappointments in your life and that therefore you should eat Trash Food or eat when you are not hungry in order to immediately feel better," he says. "But Sane Adult will silence her, telling her that everyone struggles with problems. You do not have to eat down your problems. By repeatedly listening to your Sane Adult, you will *acquire an escape from overeating.*"

I do not see any escape hatch *yet.*

"Young Jackie, nothing can make you give in to Trash Food or give in to eating when you are not a three in hunger, if you think out of your Sane Adult mind. Of course, your Demanding Child will give you every reason in the world to give in, because she is only interested in immediate gratification. Your ability to tap into your Sane Adult's thinking gives you an incredible form of power. Hard things exist in life, such as annoying coworkers, health issues, car accidents, financial setbacks, being misunderstood, people you love making wrong choices, and possibly being a victim of a crime. Indeed, these are serious setbacks and highly unwanted situations. In the midst of great adversity, your Demanding Child will especially roar and try to convince you that these situations are special and that you should therefore give yourself a food treat to make yourself feel better. Ridiculous. *Even in the midst of great adversity, you can still ditch sweets and starches, plan, shop, and prep, and wait until you are a three to eat. You have a choice how to respond* to any situation. Either you listen to your Demanding Child, who is responsible for your last thirteen years of suffering with your weight, *or* you listen to your Sane Adult, knowing that medicating your adversity or low mood with food will not make your trial go away and will only keep you from one of your current Top Four Life Goals. Many women are unnecessarily slaves to the instincts and impulses of the Demanding Child. You do not have to be. You never lose the freedom to choose. In every situation, you can let your Sane Adult be in charge of your decisions. You are not powerless at all, but incredibly powerful."

Powerful? He is talking about the wrong chick. I'm a wet noodle.

"Never will there be a season of life where all goes completely smooth," he says. "Just when you think you have got one set of problems solved, another set rear its ugly head. Things will crash down around you. People will rattle you; unpleasant situations will feel like they might swallow you. This is *normal* life, and your Demanding Child will react by wanting to eat to temporarily distract herself from the uncomfortableness. This is a repeated—and repeated—and repeated pattern, and it has robbed you of living your life in a thin body."

I keep thinking that a smooth, problem-free life is right around the river bend and *then* I will get thin.

"You choose your thoughts, Young Jackie. You can choose to look at cheesecake as pleasure, delight, fantasy, and escape. Or you look at cheesecake as the stealer of your dreams, as the bringer of cancer, heart attacks, wide hips, sluggish mind, and a discouraging attitude. Your Sane Adult will tell you that cheesecake—and other sugary cohorts—rob and diminish the enjoyment of your very life, *not add to it. What we tell ourselves about the cheesecake determines our choice whether to eat it or not.* You have leverage you do not know you had. You are not a victim."

I feel like a victim.

"Life can be frustrating, but the time for using food to medicate discomfort and to invoke stimulation and entertainment is past. *You now eat for nutrition and hunger.* Anything else your Demanding Child throws at you is ludicrous."

"But Genie, I was not born with natural willpower."

"Eating is not about willpower," he says. "If you were held captive by a terrorist, and he said he would cut off your arm if you ate the pie in front of you, would you have any trouble finding willpower? None. Why? *Because thoughts and beliefs drive actions.* You believe your arm is worth more than the pie. But when you look at that same pie at a dinner party, you listen to your Demanding Child say, 'Oh, I want some. That looks so delish, and everybody else gets to enjoy some. Anyhow, my life is stressful, and I am tired, and this will make me feel better.' That is only your Demanding Child and her self-pity. That is her entitlement saying that she is too important to have to withstand the normal stress of trials that are common to every human. Eating down stress is your Demanding Child saying that she will not tolerate *not having things go her way.* You see, *losing weight is not really about willpower.* It is about seeing that your *thoughts drive your decisions* regarding whether you are going to eat or not."

I will have to take some time to process this. My previous mentality is being dynamited.

"Another lie of your Demanding Child is that more is desirable. The truth is *enough* is desirable and *more* makes you fat and depressed. 'Enough is as good as a feast,' remember? You can learn to stop yourself after a small portion. Food does not have a magic power that says, 'Eat!' No, the thoughts of your Demanding Child are driving you to want the immediate comfort and entertainment. What make you fat are your *thoughts* that demand to be comforted and entertained right now. You can learn to *think* differently than this."

Well, I cannot learn that today.

"It is good if you almost mock your Demanding Child, laughing at her powerless attempts to get you to eat outside the *Skinny School* lessons. Why, your Demanding Child does not even get a vote. Would you let a real demanding child, such as a rude nephew, come to your house and paint your walls lime green? Of course you would not. A demanding nephew is not in charge. But your Demanding Child likes to act like she is in charge, throwing herself on the floor with her tantrums and demands. Your Sane Adult, your will to choose, is in control and makes all of your final decisions. The decisions to plan, to shop, to prep, to throw out Trash Food, to exercise early in the day while you still feel good, to ditch sweets and starches, and to wait until you are a three to eat…These are the money."[7]

Exercise? *Did he say* exercise? We have not talked about exercise before. I should have known this program was going to get harder.

"This battle with your weight is won by a pit bull tenacity that refuses to consider giving in to the spoiled Demanding Child who has ruined things long enough," he says. "Your Sane Adult knows that you must get rid of that ugly self-pity where you feel sorry for yourself. It is a privilege to live as a human, and it is a necessity to learn to shut up your Demanding Child so you can achieve your true goals."

I sort of thought that food was one friend I had to comfort and entertainment me, but now, he says I need to only eat for nutrition and hunger. I am afraid this is going to be a long and winding road.

"You have assigned the wrong meaning to food in your life," he continues. "Your Demanding Child has erroneously told you food is zest, stimulation, color, comfort, and entertainment. The truth is that food is merely pleasant-tasting nutrition. Focus on the Miraculous Threesome: Ditch, Plan, Wait. Your Sane Adult can choose to make these choices all day long, plodding through each day, returning again and again to these one-two-three rules."

This is not nearly as easy as he proposes.

"For years, the debate has raged between your Demanding Child and your Sane Adult. It is time to end that debate and instead to dig a grave for your Demanding Child. You are *missing out on the great joy of self-mastery.*

---

7 Lesson Eight is about a clean environment and Lesson Nine is on exercise.

When your Demanding Child says, 'You should eat that,' the answer from your Sane Adult is, 'No. Eating Trash Food and eating when I am not hungry do not get me what I truly want. I am frumpy and chubby *exactly because of those two issues*. I will no longer let them rob me of a thin body.'"

"Genie, this is overwhelming and complicated," I plead. I mean, this is a total 180 for me.

"It is not complicated, Young Jackie. Your eating problem is simple. You have three and only three issues to overcome. One, you eat the wrong food, Trash Food. Two, you eat good food, but you eat when you are not truly hungry. And three, you are hungry, eat the right food, but do not stop when you have had enough—you eat past a five. That is not complicated but extremely simple. Not easy, but simple."

At least he admits it is not easy.

"Again, the secret is *your mind, your thoughts*," he says. "When you see those three issues as the only culprits that are keeping you from the thin body you desire, you can come up with the strength to choose."

Thinking that *these one-two-three rules are all that stand between me and size six jeans* makes me feel a little dizzy. Is he possibly right?

"I admit you are giving up something you enjoy, a pleasurable taste experience and a quick way to dial down the emotional intensity of a situation. And we will discuss nonfood ways to dial down your emotions in Lesson Seven. But you must remember that thinness and health are a current Top Four Life Goal to you. The human experience includes learning to overcome obstacles. Foregoing immediate pleasure to acquire a current Top Four Life Goal is a necessary lesson for all humans."

Instead of taking AP calculus in school, I should have taken this course.

"I want to discuss another idea that will motivate you to choose well," he says. "Consider how good you feel when you eat well, and consider how discouraged you feel when you give in to your Demanding Child."

"Yes," I say, "after I give in to my Demanding Child, I fall into a blue funk."

"The Demanding Child part of your brain does not want you to remember this," he says. "She wants pleasure right now. Your Sane Adult knows that when you eat right, you feel more energized and happy. Your Sane Adult also knows that you later experience suffering when you go off your program. However, your Demanding Child comes in, and she feels like she handcuffs and gags the Sane Adult. But that is not true. Your Sane Adult has merely not been trained to step up and to debate the Demanding Child."

Uh, my brain parts are going to debate each other? This sounds a little quirky.

"Often you will find that when you eat and reach a five in fullness, you will hear your Demanding Child say, 'I would like a little more, please.' It will always be in a sweet voice that the Demanding Child speaks, as that is part of the manipulation. The voice is soft and acts like it has your best interests at heart. But move over and address your Sane Adult. Ask Sane Adult what she thinks about it. You truly are accessing another brain lobe, the one that thinks with logic. Your Sane Adult will tell you, 'You ate an appropriate amount to get to a five in fullness, and you are no longer hungry. This is a manipulation of your Demanding Child to get more pleasure, even though she has had enough.' Just hearing Your Sane Adult speak will give you the strength to walk away from your Demanding Child and get busy with something else. But you have to access your Sane Adult. You have to intentionally move into another part of your brain."

Now he thinks he is a neurologist.

"Your Sane Adult needs to remember that *the source of your suffering from your weight problem is from all the immediate gratification that the Demanding Child has talked you into.* Frumpiness is the result of listening to your Demanding Child over the years."

And I thought my Demanding Child was taking care of me.

"Your Demanding Child will say, 'It is so sad how I have to deprive myself.' But move into Sane Adult. Ask her opinion. She will say, 'No one gets everything in life. We all know we must give up *some* things to get *better* things. You have decided to give up sweets, starches, and seconds so you can instead get a thin, hard, smokin' body.'"

The thought of a thin, hard, smokin' body still seems reserved for the Evas and Rachels of the world, not for the ordinary Jackies.

"Remember, Young Jackie, this is a six-month course. By the end of this course, you will clearly hear your Demanding Child with all of her brilliant reasons why you should eat off your *Skinny School* plan, and you will be able to debunk every one of them."

Promises, promises.

"Demanding Child will use all of her reasons why you should engage in immediate gratification and eat off your plan. But Sane Adult can stop that whining by remembering that you have given in to your Demanding Child for years, and it never got you what you really, deeply wanted."

Oh, if only I could count on this. Because, if this is true—oh, if this is possibly true—then I see how I might, for the first time, be able to resist eating off my plan. I would have a *strategy to win those conversations that battle each other in my mind!*

"This is simply a skill to learn, Young Jackie. You will not master this overnight. But my *Skinny School* students of the past have mastered this thinking. It is truly one of the hugest secrets in the world of skinniness."

Is it possible I might have found the golden key to escape fat prison?

"You may have heard others say they have 'flipped a switch' or they 'will never go back to eating as before.' All they mean is that they have finally learned that *eating for comfort and pleasure is a ruse;* the true goodness is in *ditching Trash Food, planning beautiful, legitimate food to have ready to eat, and waiting until you are a three to eat.*"

The Miraculous Threesome: Ditch, Plan, Wait. Should I make a poster of those rules and put them on my bathroom mirror?

"What you must understand is that you have a mind-set in concrete right now that tells you that you can eat what and when you want and *still be thin.* It is a lie. You either decide that you will continue to eat like you have been, or you make a decision to forgo some treats in life as far as food. Life is rich and full of pleasure, like the pleasure of seeing, the pleasure of hearing, the pleasure of smelling, the pleasure of reading, the pleasure of learning, the pleasure of creating…so many fabulous pleasures to embrace. But somehow, you have focused on the pleasure of taste alone. You do not have to give up that pleasure, but to be thin, you certainly have to restrict it."

"Can you give me some concrete examples of what I say to my Demanding Child when she appears, Genie?" This is as foreign to me as nuclear physics. Actually, I know more about nuclear physics than this.

"If your Demanding Child suggests to you, 'That Trash Food looks so tasty, and you need a little reward since you have been working very hard,' then write that sentence down in your Ruby Journal on List 5: 'Repeated Schemes My Demanding Child Uses.' Next to this, write down a possible response of your Sane Adult, such as, 'You want thinness more than a short-lived taste experience—which you have already tried a zillion times and it did not get you what you wanted. Remember, you have wanted thinness with an intensity, a fervor, and a passion for thirteen years.' Young Jackie, it is these twenty or so individual battles with your Demanding Child that you must overcome in order to control your weight. Get some veggies out of your Quart Bags and a glass of herbal tea, and get your mind on something else, possibly reading something interesting on the web."

I keep forgetting about having those Quart Bags around.

"Here is another example," he says. "Suppose you have a plan for the day of what you are going to eat when you are truly hungry. A neighbor knocks on your door and has baked you fresh brownies. You thank her and carry the brownies to the kitchen. Now, the clanging debate begins. Your Sane Adult will say, 'Oh dear, those are not on my plan. I should not eat these.' And then your Demanding Child will say, 'It will hurt your neighbor's feelings if you do not eat them. Just have one. Besides, it is a shame to waste those beautiful brownies.' "

Ha-ha...that is exactly the conversation that my brain would have.

"Your Demanding Child always wants what is most pleasurable at the moment," he says. "She has no thought about what is good for you long-term. You must have your antennas up and listen for her demands. They will always be cradled in terms of 'enjoy it right now' and 'immediate gratification.' Once you start listening for her manipulation, you can tear her mask off."

What ludicrous internal conversations I have.

"Let's try this together," he proposes. "Write down in your Ruby Journal the scenario of your Demanding Child whispering to you to enjoy a brownie right now. Then on the right, answer how your Sane Adult feels about this request of your Demanding Child."

I sit in silence for a minute.

"I do not know what to write, Genie," I say. I guess I am only smart in certain areas.

"All right, I will help you on this one," he says. "Here is what your Sane Adult would want to say, if you ask her: 'I, your Sane Adult, know that you will not eat just one bite, and that this is a trick of the Demanding Child. Also, this is how the floodgates open, when you say you are going to just taste it. You end up eating a little more and a little more and then going Hog Wild. I, your Sane Adult, also know that this is Trash Food and that it does not nourish your body. Please do not listen to your Demanding Child. She is only interested in what is comfortable and pleasurable at this moment. What you really want is long-term thinness, and that is achieved by staying on your plan."

"How could I ever figure all this out, Genie? I will never get all this." Valedictorian or not, this is difficult stuff.

"Of course you will get this," he says. "Another example that might occur is during dinner when you simply want seconds. Your Demanding Child will say something to you in your own voice like, 'It is sad that I only get one serving. Poor me. I have so many trials, and that extra serving would taste so yummy.'"

Laughing again, I realize that this is the exact conversation I would have in my thoughts.

"Immediately access your Sane Adult," he says. "Your Sane Adult will say, 'I am not going to eat seconds although it would be tasty. I want something more, and that is thinness. I do love pleasure though, and therefore I will make myself some herbal chocolate tea or some raspberry tea, sweetened with Stevia. I will find other ways to enjoy or calm myself.'"

I like that sentence: *I can find other ways to entertain and soothe myself.*

"Let us explore another example," he continues. "Suppose it is after dinner and you ate an appropriate dinner, stopping at a five. There is an ad on TV that makes you want to get the ice cream out of your freezer, even though you are not hungry. You are eating for entertainment or self-soothing at this point. But your Demanding Child says to you in your own voice, 'That ice cream in the fridge would be creamy and tasty right now. A couple tablespoons will not derail my diet. Anyhow, I walked two miles today, so I can eat a little extra.'"

How does he have access to my thoughts? Anyhow, this time I think I might have an idea how to handle this scenario. I say, "I would then access my Sane Adult and ask her what she thinks. My Sane Adult would say, 'Jackie, you are not hungry. You just want to entertain and soothe yourself. That ice cream will open the floodgates, and you will not stick to one or two bites. You never do. Do not be fooled by your Demanding Child for immediate pleasure. Stick to your plan. That is how to get thin. And thin is what you really want. That desire is only your Demanding Child wanting instant gratification.'"

"Bravo!" he yells, pumping the air with his fist. "That is exactly what you would say to debate your Demanding Child. When you can access your Sane Adult like this, you can then strip the power from your Demanding Child."

By George, I think I've got it.

"Indulging your Demanding Child is never a good decision for a Champion," he says. *"Now is the time to decide that no one, no schedule, no adversity, no celebration, no special event will pull you off track.* Enter the No Excuse Zone, and do not even let your mind toy with going off your plan. This is a current Top Four Life Goal for you, and it is time you went after it with everything in you. This hurdle of your weight has beaten you down for years. It is time to take back the ground. The *Skinny School* lessons are the path out of the dungeon."

A fat dungeon, a dark dungeon, a sad dungeon.

"It is your birthday, you are on vacation, it is the weekend, you have had a hard day, you need a reward, you are tired, it is a holiday season—the excuses of your Demanding Child are infinite. However, your answer to Demanding Child's request to eat Trash Food or to eat when you are not physically hungry is, 'No, I will stick to the *Skinny School* rules—Ditch, Plan, Wait—until I reach Goal A. Then I will only engage in Planned Cheating,' which, by the way, we will discuss in the future in Lesson Twenty-Two."

At least there is hope for some allowed cheating in the future. I hope I get to go crazy and eat unlimited amounts of yummy stuff.

"There will be a time in the near future," he says, "when you will not succumb to the Demanding Child's pleads. After the moment passes, you will say to yourself, 'Wow, I am so proud of myself for not doing the easy thing but doing the thing that gets me what I want most: thinness!' You will find that self-mastery bring you much joy."

Oh, happy day.

"And someday soon," he says, "you will be out socializing, and others who are chubby will be eating dessert and other Trash Food, and you will say to yourself, 'They do not have the secrets to get out of Food Prison. That is sad. Maybe someday I can help them.'"

Sure. Soon...like in the next millennium.

"I know your thinking is not there yet, but it is coming," he says. "You and you alone are responsible for training your mind to think like this. That is why I repeatedly ask you to daily bathe your mind with motivation and the right thoughts from your Sane Adult, written down in your Ruby Journal, or else the deep grooves and habits of your Demanding Child will continue to rule. The escape from Food Horrorville is in changing *how you think*."

Living in Food Horrorville is true, but this whole escape thing is still very questionable.

"There is a recipe of Genie Quiche in your fridge," he says, and with that, he dissolves into the atmosphere. This is like *Star Trek*. Beam me up, Scottie.

Pulling into my apartment complex, I notice a package from UPS for me from Dubai. Opening the package, I discover a beautiful bracelet. Could these little stones be real diamonds? Dating Brandon and getting diamond bracelets sure beats the occasional CD that Robert would give me (which would always be bands Robert liked, anyhow.) Putting the bracelet back in the box, I notice that the kitchen is an absolute wreck. Then Tory walks out of her bedroom with her keys, getting ready to leave, wearing my new shoes!

She is caught red-handed, and we both just stare at each other. Another month's rent is due, and she still has not paid last month's. "Tory!" I say with annoyance in my voice.

"I didn't have any other shoes to match, and I was in a hurry," she whined.

"Tory, your feet are actually a size bigger than mine, so you will stretch my shoes. I'm sorry, but I'm going to have to ask you not to wear them," I say, simmering right at the boiling point. I begin to mention the rent and the dishes, but she bursts out crying.

"Oh, what will I wear?" she pleads and runs off to her room and slams the door. As I walk by her door on the way to my room, I hear her talking to her mom on the phone.

"Miss Chubby is so selfish with everything. She is always getting on me for everything!" she cries to her mom.

This roommate eviction is looong overdue. Indeed! Miss Chubby!

Gosh, my life is miserable right now. But my Sane Adult will not let me medicate this feeling of being upset with Trash Food. Gee, what should I do instead? Grabbing some herbal tea and some veggies from my Quart Bags, I undress. A hot bath and a Calvin and Hobbes comic book might be just the thing I need to calm down.

The nonnegotiables in *Skinny School* so far are:

1. I expect to work like a Champion to retrain my mind since this is a current Top Four Life Goal.
2. Ditching sweets and starches is not optional if I want to overhaul my metabolism. I am to track my sugar/carb grams as well as my calories. I focus on all the beautiful, delicious food *I get to eat* instead of what I must not eat.
3. Planning and prepping are the secrets Champions use to conquer goals. I must daily make Quart Bags.
4. Hunger is my friend, and waiting until I am truly hungry and quitting before I am full are nonnegotiable. Tracking my hunger is imperative and will expose how I deceive myself with wanting to eat for self-soothing and entertainment.

5. By listing the schemes of Demanding Child in my Ruby Journal and accessing how my Sane Adult really feels, I can dismantle the Demanding Child's tricks, one by one.

Lesson 6

Don't Waste Failure

Friday, August 29   *Weight: 169*   *Pounds lost: 6*   *Still to lose: 39*

The Genie is right that I am much happier when I stay on my program. That old feeling of disgust and self-incrimination is horrible, and this new feeling of emotional freedom is invigorating instead. As the Genie reminded me, I feel like a different person when I am following the *Skinny School* program. I need to write that down in my Ruby Journal for motivation to not go off my plan.

Mrs. Lyle, a client, is in Zach's office and is upset over the monetary negotiations of her case. Having worked with Attorney Fortwright on many settlements that are very similar to Mrs. Lyle's case, I can tell Mrs. Lyle is being extremely unreasonable. Yes, her arm got broken in the accident, but she wants tens of thousands of dollars for her pain and suffering, and no insurance company is going to get close to that. Mrs. Lyle leaves rather abruptly, not getting the satisfaction she wanted from Zach.

It is almost lunchtime and since I did not pack my lunch, I get ready to leave to go buy a salad at Whole Foods. Sticking my head in Zach's office, I ask, "Would you like me to pick up something for you at Whole Foods, or did you lose your appetite after that confrontation with Mrs. Lyle?"

The stress is written all over Zach's face. Difficult clients are definitely not a fun part of his job. "After that confrontation, I completely lost *all* of my appetite," he says.

"Mrs. Lyle was ridiculously unreasonable, Zach. I heard it all from my desk. Why, you have negotiated down her medical bills, and also you are taking a cut in your fee to make her happy, and it is still not enough for her. That is a great settlement you are getting, but she wants the moon. You cannot let people who are unreasonable make you feel bad. You are an amazing lawyer, Zach. She is a little on the crazy side, if you ask me."

Zach looks at me, stone faced. Maybe I should stick to typing and not try to be Dr. Phil.

"I appreciate that, Jackie." No smile, but he looks a little less upset. I turn to leave, and he says, "Hey, my appetite just returned. How about bringing me a cheese pizza?" Pizza is not on my *Skinny School* program, but normal people like Zach can eat a few carbs.

Turning back around, I notice all of the previous stress on his face is completely gone. He looks normal again. "By the way, I am treating both of us today," he says, as he reaches for his wallet to get his Visa. "It is the least I can do for the free counseling." He is teasing me, but he is also serious. He appreciated what I said.

I wave the Visa in the air. "I am not sure you should trust me with this Visa, Zach. There is a sale going on at Macy's, and it is right next door to Whole Foods."

Again, he slightly grins. "I feel pretty good about trusting you with just about *everything*, Jackie." He is still staring at me with a faint smile.

Wow. I am not sure what to do with that. That was pretty nice. I mean, that was *really* nice. Zach just said he feels good about trusting me with just about *everything*. Walking out of the office, I can feel that compliment warming my entire inner being. Zach trusts me. And he wanted to tell me. I realize again how the right words *from the right person* have a gargantuan effect on a person's psyche. That compliment was like pouring a dose of happiness all over my brain.

Walking into Whole Foods, I order Zach's pizza and then begin thinking about my next brief assignment. Ideas start downloading themselves from the cosmos. This happens to me, where ideas start flowing in a crazy stream. I do not have my iPad with me, but I do have a legal pad in my trunk, so I return to my car to fish it out. Before I get my salad, I sit down and go to town for about fifteen minutes, writing down ideas, an outline, and good sentences to use. I love when I am in the zone. These ideas for Zach's brief are especially good. After I type them up at the office, I will show them to Zach.

The word has traveled around the office how I can write briefs, how caught up Zach is on his work, and what a wiz I am. I admit it—I like it when others think I am brainy. This is maybe my imagination, but it seems everybody treats me a little nicer now that I am the *smart* fat girl.

Walking into the break room when I get back to the office, I set down my purse and the legal pad where I recorded five pages of notes so I can get an afternoon cup of coffee. I leave everything in the break room for a second while I deliver Zach's cheese pizza to him.

Returning to the break room, there is my legal pad with slushy coffee grinds all over it. Eva is standing there with the coffee grinds basket, like she got caught with her hand in the cookie jar.

"My notes!" I say as I quickly grab them, pouring the coffee grinds in the trash, trying to salvage my notes. Too late. The ink is smeared and the notes are gone forever.

In the most matter-of-fact voice, Eva says, "I was about to spill the grinds on my new skirt, so I had to drop them somewhere."

Are you kidding me? So she drops them on someone's notes?

"Those were my notes for my brief for Zach," I say.

"A brief for Zach is very important," she says, with almost snide sarcasm in her voice. She would not do this on purpose, would she? Attorney Simpson walks in the room to get his afternoon coffee, says a bright hello to me, and before I can even respond, Eva begins to tell him how her car is not working right and asks him where she should take it to get repaired. I am ignored like I am a pile of coffee grinds. Daddy and daughter are talking about her little sports car and Huge Heifer Jackie and her stained notes are ignored. I walk to my desk to try to calm down.

Trying to recreate my thoughts from my notes, I feel very offended. Mistreated. Angry. Attorney Simpson again walks by my desk in his obvious thousand-dollar suit on his way into Zach's office. "Jackie, what a pretty red scarf!" he says. He is often nicey-nice, dropping compliments here and there. A little twitch inside of me warns me to not fully trust him, but maybe, I think, that is just my problem of being too suspicious of everybody.

Shutting the door behind him, Attorney Simpson begins to talk in a low voice to Zach. Although I am still worked up from Eva's inconsiderate actions, I am now more interested in why Attorney Simpson would shut the door. Hardly anyone shuts their door in this firm. Attorney Simpson goes into Zach's office all the time to talk, but he never has shut the door before. I am not proud of what I do next, but I do it anyhow. The file cabinet is right next to Zach's door, so I decide that if I file right now, I might be able to hear what Attorney Simpson is saying to Zach. Quickly, I walk over to the file cabinet.

"Zach, what do you think about the idea of Jackie training Eva to be a legal assistant?" Attorney Simpson asks Zach.

There is a pause. A long one. I know Zach thinks it is a bad idea. Zach asks, "For you, sir? Is she training Eva for you?"

Another pause. Another long pause.

"Actually, I was thinking Jackie could train Eva for you, Zach," Attorney Simpson says.

What? I think. Zach does not want Miss Pea Brain working for him! Besides, *I* work for Zach.

"I have got Jackie, sir, and she is doing an amazing job for me," Zach respectfully says.

"That is the other thing I wanted to talk to you about, "he says. "I am thinking of promoting Jackie to *executive* legal assistant, paying her ten thousand dollars more a year, and using her for *my* assistant."

Oh, my gosh! No. No! I do not want to be his assistant. Money or no money. Title or no title. And I do not want to train Eva to be Zach's assistant, which is a ridiculous joke anyways—she can hardly spell—and I do not want to give up smelling Zach's cologne and looking at his white crisp starched shirts every morning.

"Now, Zach, if you decide you must keep Jackie," Attorney Simpson continues, "that is fine, but then she will not get the raise or the new title. But I will not tell her. That will be your decision. But the opportunity is available to her."

"With all respect, sir," Zach says, "Eva is untrained, and Jackie is probably the best assistant in town."

"I know, my boy, I know," Attorney Simpson says, like it is the easiest problem in the world to solve. "Jackie will train Eva and teach her all she knows. Eva just needs a little grooming."

A little grooming! More like a brain transplant. Oh, sure, that is easy. I will just plug my brain—that has been drenched with law for the last five years—and download everything into Numbskull Eva's brain. Easy. Just so easy.

Zach is speechless.

"Well, think about it and let me know," Attorney Simpson says.

"I am extremely reluctant to give up Jackie," Zach pleads again.

"I understand, but then Jackie will miss out on the promotion and the raise," he says, appealing to Zach's moral code to not limit another's progress and benefit. I scurry back to my desk before I get caught eavesdropping.

Just as I sit down, Attorney Simpson steps out of Zach's office. Again he smiles widely and says, "Jackie, we are certainly pleased with your work," and leaves.

So now I get it. If Zach gives me up, I get a ten-thousand-dollar-a-year raise, but he gets high-fashion-low-brain Eva. But if he keeps me, I do not get the raise. Being a person of integrity, Zach wouldn't selfishly hold me back from what seems to be an obvious promotion. But then, he is stuck with Eva.

I do not want a raise. Or a promotion. I like being right here, ten yards from Zach's desk, hearing his voice on the phone all day long, taking pictures with him, stopping for a salad with salmon with him. No. No. I don't want to go anywhere.

Zach comes out of his office and hands me some letters, not even making eye contact.

My expectations were that he would give me a kind, caring look, suggesting that he is struggling with losing me as his personal assistant but that he has to give me up because that is the best thing for me. He does not even look at me. Maybe he feels guilty that he is going to keep me—which means I will not get the raise.

Just before he walks back into his office, he turns and says, "The Whitehorn brief is due in three weeks, just to remind you. And the Applegate brief is due in six weeks." He does not smile and walks back to his desk.

Oh, my gosh! He is going to keep me! He is going to keep me from that ten-thousand-dollar raise, just so I will write his stupid briefs. Yes, he can treat me to a stupid Whole Foods salad and throw out some nice words about trusting me, but they all mean nothing. All of a sudden, I am reminded of what I mean to Zach. *Why, I am just some robot who does his work, like some fancy software program.* I am a *thing*. It is nothing personal. *Jackie, wake up!* I say to myself. This is not about me personally. It is about the work I grind out. He has a girlfriend, and I am *the help. The help*, Jackie. That is all you are.

Even though a second ago I wanted Zach to keep me so I could smell his cologne every morning, now I am mad that he is keeping me, obviously demonstrating that *his* interests are more important than *mine*. What an idiot I am.

Tonight is the Employee Appreciation Dinner, and I want to stay home alone and eat Trash Food, medicating all my discouragement. What a true dunce I am. Just because I am book smart and capable, I somehow thought that would wedge me into Zach's mind and heart. Such a downright loser I am. I am a *thing*, a disposable, replaceable machine that is well oiled and greased, aiding Zach in his goals. How smooth he is, buttering me all up with those nice words and that Visa.

Gathering my purse and things, I think I may somehow try to get that executive legal assistant job myself and get that ten-grand raise. Hmpf! Then I will laugh as Zach struggles with Anorexia Eva and her misspellings.

Anyhow, I could use the ten grand. Going to law school is not cheap. And besides, Zach is getting ready to get engaged, and I do not want to be near him when Rachel is coming in the office every day, showing him china patterns and talking about rose bouquets and black-and-white photography. I will be better off as Attorney Simpson's assistant anyhow, away from Zach and Rachel's life.

Getting up to leave, I hear Zach call from his desk, "See you in a couple of hours. Save me a seat by you, okay?"

Can you believe it? He is acting like everything is cool, like we are the Dynamic Duo. Ha! We will see about that.

"I might be a few minutes late," he says. "I need to have a meeting with Attorney Simpson."

Caught in the moment without a comeback, I simply say, "Okay," and exit. Of course! He needs to tell Attorney Simpson he is keeping me for himself because I am his little work grinder.

How stupid of me, I realize again, to want to hang around Zach. His engagement is going to be sooner rather than later, and then, if I am still his assistant, I will have to be around Rachel and her bridesmaid-luncheons talk and all that hoopla. This is a J-O-B. It is not about *me*—it is about the work I produce. How ridiculous for me to keep expecting these coworkers to actually care about *me*. I am a merely a dollar sign.

I have got to get a life. My job has taken on meaning that it should not, with me wanting others to care about me and like me. I will go home, shower and shampoo, and look the best I can tonight, but then I will ignore Zach the whole night. I will quit trying to get blood out of that turnip.

Even though I am only down six pounds, it feels like more. I think of the outfit I have bought for tonight. The navy dress I bought is soft, and the ruffles around the neck are flattering. I do feel pretty and confident in it. So maybe I will have a good time tonight and ignore Mr. Zach Boltz, who could care less if I live or die—just so long as I crank out his work.

Arriving home, I open the fridge before I get in the shower. Nothing much in there, as I forgot to make my Quart Bags, so I open the pantry. In the back are some chocolate chips that I used to eat that I forgot to throw away. Chocolate is one of those foods that has antioxidants, isn't it? Don't I need some after this war zone at work? I am going to dinner in an hour, so I will only eat three or four. Oooh, these are good. Three or four more will not hurt me. Heck, I will just finish the bag so they do not sit here and torture me.

After I eat all the chocolate chips, I realize I shouldn't have. Oh well, now that I have blown it, I might as well eat all I want. Finding an unopened bag of chocolate-covered almonds, I wolf them down. And then I dive into a bag of cookies.

Finally feeling full, I hear the band practicing at the nearby high school for their first Friday night football game. The music reminds me of when I was in high school. I remember watching all the skinny girls with their new skinny jeans tucked inside their boots, looking like one long piece of rope. And then there was me, trying to look hip, tucking my over-sized jeans into my expensive Calvin Klein boots, trying to keep up and to feel included. I was fine in the stands with the girls during the game, as we all cheered and yelled. But when the game was over, all the skinny girls went down on the field to talk to their boyfriends. I remember desperately looking around, trying to find someone to talk to so I wouldn't be alone. Everyone was nice to me, of course, but when it was time to pair up, I was paired with Caitlin, an unattractive girl who was five foot eleven and who had as much trouble as me attracting cute guys. Freddy, a likeable and funny boy who was very short and had a lot of acne, always hung around, wanting to know if I wanted to go with him to McAlisters to get a sandwich. That is the best I could do in high school, Freddy Sammons. I was in the top one percent in academics. But all I could score with the guys was Freddy Sammons.

Often, I made excuses not to join everyone and then would drive through Jack in the Box and order the works. Feeling stuffed, I would then not focus on how sad I was about the lack of interest from the cute guys. Instead, I would focus on my despicable weight, my binge eating, and my disgust with myself.

Getting into the shower, I'm overwhelmed by a similar feeling of that high school despair, thinking of Zach using me and then about how I am never going to lose weight because I keep giving in to Trash Food. My Demanding Child will never be stopped. Even after that sermon on my Demanding Child and Sane Adult, I still cannot resist Trash Food.

Beginning to apply my makeup, I wonder if there is any way I could bail on tonight. **Surprisingly, the Genie appears in my bathroom.** Oh, dear. This is not a good time for another lesson. At least I have on a robe.

"Good evening, Young Jackie. Now that you are beginning to understand the shenanigans of your Demanding Child, much insight will become available to you. You now know that Demanding Child is always lurking in the shadows, trying to press you for immediate gratification with no thought of your actual goals. Today we will learn about two important activities to deactivate many of Demanding Child's ploys."

"I hope you have something else to help me, Genie, because I am not doing too well in your *Skinny School* program," I admit. *Not doing too well* is a gross understatement.

"You are doing fine," he says. "I told you that the 'click' and 'flipping of the switch' probably would not appear until Lesson Seven."

I thought the last lesson was supposed to flip the switch.

"The normal human pattern," says the Genie, "is *try, fail, then give up*. But there is a much better pattern available. It is *try, fail, explore why you failed, learn from it, and try again*. Humans are going to have failure. But *do not waste the valuable learning that failure can bring you*. If you recognize your normal pattern and then overlay the correct pattern, you can eventually figure out how to solve a problem."

I hate failure, and I will never be able to learn from my insanity eating.

"I want to discuss what to do when you fail on your *Skinny School* program," the Genie begins.

I frown. He must have been watching my recent escapade in the kitchen from the cosmos.

"Today, I want to change how you think about failure forever," he says.

The way I feel about failure is that it defines me, and I am a loser with a capital *L*.

"Failure happens to all humans," he says. "What is different among humans, though, is how they respond to failure."

I respond by eating *even more* to medicate my failure—thus creating *more* failure.

"Did you know that failure can be a good thing?" he asks.

Sometimes he says stupid stuff, but saying that failure is good must be among the stupidest.

"Failure can show you what does not work, and if you are savvy, you can take this information and use it to help you reach your goals," he says. "As I have said before, you do not have two thousand potholes you step in that derail you in your *Skinny School* program. You have about twenty. If you will list each of the ways your Demanding Child trips you up in your Ruby Journal—List 5: 'Repeated Schemes My Demanding Child Uses'—and then write the corresponding and wise thoughts of your Sane Adult, you will be more and more prepared to handle the same trip-up the next time."

I do not think anyone or anything can help me, the loser of the century.

"Open your Ruby Journal, and let's add what just happened to List Five."

I would rather erase that from my memory.

"What I want you to do is to write how Sane Adult should have talked to Demanding Child at that moment."

Should have. But did not.

"When you reread this list of potholes regularly, you strip power from your Demanding Child's tactics. Eventually, your Demanding Child will run out of schemes."

Right. I believe that. Just like Prince Harry is trying right now to get my number.

"Young Jackie, the human experience is full of failure. You must learn how to respond to failure. You can feel discouraged when you fail, or instead, you can choose to record your failure, find alternate Sane Adult thoughts, and then use the information to help you make better choices in the future. *Do not waste failure; embrace it, evaluate it, learn from it.*"

Embrace it? He acts like failure is some resource, like gold or silver.

"Failure can be your friend," he says. "And if you will embrace and explore the failure, you will discover hidden truths and opportunities in failure. Because failure feels painful to humans, they run from it, medicate it, and try to ignore it. But the best way to deal with failure is, again, to record it, evaluate why it happened, and to consider what your Sane Adult *should have thought* at that moment. Frequently rereading this list enables you to eventually not step in the same potholes."

Large potholes. Many potholes. Deep potholes.

"Do you see how important your Ruby Journal is?" he asks. "This is where you accumulate your new thought. Washing your brain with your new thought will begin to make new neural pathways in your brain. Eventually, like a schoolyard path that is no longer used, your old thoughts and brain paths will be overridden with your new ways to think."

I only have sixty to seventy more years to live, not nearly long enough to override my previous neural pathways.

"When you fail, like a few moments ago," he says, "write it down, evaluate the failure—what tripped you up?—figure out what Sane Adult wanted you to think, and then there is something else very important to do after that."

Oh, no. He wants me to run five or six miles to make up for the calories.

"Draw a line in the sand and forget it," he says. "Regrets are only useful when you learn from them. You can waste untold time and energy thinking about regrets and failure. Do not do that. Look at your day and see what you need to do. Then begin to tackle the tasks on your day's list, refusing to think about your failure anymore. Failure can be an instrument for greater insight, or failure can keep you discouraged and paralyzed in a ditch."

Paralyzed in a ditch. Check.

"Your Demanding Child has some strongly ingrained habits in your life," he says. "You will not conquer her in a day. The new pattern is try, fail, and learn. Try again, fail, and learn some more. And before long you will alert your Sane Adult how to steer clear of the Demanding Child's potholes."

I'm sick of trying. I'm sick of failing.

"You may have failed in the past, but that is not a predictor of the future," he says. "You can now make other choices. You can use your past failure, not merely to beat yourself up, but to learn and to go in another direction. That is one of the glorious things about a human being: *Humans can decide to change.*"

I want to change. I need to change.

"Although Demanding Child seemed like a friend in the past, she is actually more like a friend who is nice and wants to hang around so she can steal your boyfriend."

I hate those types of girls.

"The activities that we will discuss today are more work, Young Jackie, and therefore, you will initially resist them. Again I want to remind you that Champions work for their current Top Four Life Goals. Do not begrudge assignments that are engineered to change how you think. These assignments are not lifetime assignments but are very important for now while we are reprogramming your brain in *Skinny School*. Failing to comply will not give you the permanent success you desire."

Wanting something but not wanting to pay the price is a theme in my life.

"You are progressing nicely in *Skinny School*, Young Jackie. I know you want to have all the right thoughts about eating right now, but we still have many important lessons to go. You are making great headway. Be patient while we accumulate all the information you will need to rewire your brain on how to think about eating and food. I left you a recipe of Almond-Flour Fried Chicken in your fridge to eat when you are a three again," he says, and he disappears.

I ate three thousand calories a few moments ago, and he says we are making headway. He is an optimistic Genie.

Dressing quickly, I drive to the Capitol Grille, where I am led to a private room reserved for the Simpson Law Firm. Intentionally, I arrive ten minutes late, but that is a mistake. Everyone has already sat down at one long table, and there is only one seat left—and it is by Zach. Beth is sitting on the other side of the empty chair, so that is good. And of course, charming size zero Eva is flanking Zach. I can hear her babbling from here.

Although I try to slip in unobtrusively, Beth begins to *ooh* and *ahh* over my outfit. Zach is listening and turns toward me, although I don't make eye contact. "You are late," he says.

"But wasn't it worth it?" Beth asks. "Jackie, you look beautiful."

I almost say, "Beautiful if you like buffalos," but I decide not to.

Ignoring Zach, I turn to Beth and ask about Beth's favorite topic, which is her baby, Alexis. I am listening to Beth but also very mindful of what Zach is saying and doing on my other side.

When Beth takes a break in her monologue, Zach asks, "So you were late because you were primping?" I know he is just being friendly, but the friendly days are over. Mr. Charming Nice Guy! Hmpf. He sure had me fooled. Now I know when it really comes down to it, he will stab you in the back so things go well for him. I see. I see it all *very* clearly now. What a fool I have been.

Our dinner is served, and then Mr. Simpson gives a pep talk, telling everyone what a good year it has been. "You can all expect a bigger-than-usual bonus this year," he says. "And the main reason is because of the incredible work of Zach Boltz. Zach has settled some large injury cases this year, and he has made the firm a lot of money. So on behalf of the office, Zach, we thank you. And with that, you are dismissed. Thank you for coming."

Everyone claps, and Zach is his predictably humble self. What an act! Ridiculous. I could tell these people a thing or two.

Hurrying to get out the door, I feel a tug on my elbow. "What is the big rush?" I hear Zach say.

Pathetic. Pitiful. Trying to be nice but stabbing me in the back.

"I'm tired, and want to get home to go to bed," I lie.

"Okay, but I have something I want to tell you," he says. I wait. What malarkey is he going to feed me now? "You are getting a ten-thousand-dollar raise," he says.

Uh, what? I thought he was keeping me. Why did he tell me about all of those due dates of briefs if he is giving me to Attorney Simpson? I am confused.

"I am?" I ask.

"Yes, you are. I have the best assistant in the Western Hemisphere, and she should get paid more," he says.

I wait for an explanation, but he does not say anything. We just stare at each other in silence.

"Goodnight, Jackie," Zach says, and turns to leave.

What is going on? Sometimes I say too much, and this is probably one of those times, but oh, well—I really don't care.

"Zach, I am embarrassed to admit this, but I overheard the conversation between you and Attorney Simpson this afternoon. So I guess that means I will be working for him now, right?"

Zach's face is smooth, unruffled, and soft. "No, Jackie. You are not going to work for Attorney Simpson. You are still working for me. I am paying you the extra ten thousand. I didn't want you to lose the raise, but I couldn't give you up. Actually, I am getting a bargain because I get to keep you, and it only cost me ten grand." That slight grin appears on his face. I think I might faint.

I know this is not personal. I know this is not about any friendship. But still. I am wanted. And I'm being treated like I matter. I'm not only a machine that cranks out his work. I'm a human being, and Zach wants to treat me right. He wants to keep me, but he has the integrity to not let me lose the raise. I'm that important. Ten grand! Ten grand! Woo-hoo. And the best part is that Zach didn't want to lose me.

Eva walks up to our private conversation and begins, "Jackie, Daddy says you are going to train me to work for him. Will all that typing mess up my nails?"

Zach smiles again, probably as relieved that Eva is not working for him as anything.

Hearing Eva blabbing to Zach about a band downtown, I say goodnight to Beth and slip out. Ha-ha. The world can sometimes stink, but not tonight. Zach Boltz didnt want to lose me, and he is paying me out of his pocket so I don't miss the raise.

Rolling down the windows, I crank up Keith Urban's playlist and enjoy a moment...a moment of being me, chubby and all.

The nonnegotiables in *Skinny School* so far are:

1. I expect to work like a Champion to retrain my mind since this is a current Top Four Life Goal.
2. Ditching sweets and starches is not optional if I want to overhaul my metabolism. I am to track my sugar/carb grams as well as my calories. I focus on all the beautiful, delicious food I get to eat instead of what I must not eat.
3. Planning and prepping are the secrets Champions use to conquer goals. I must daily make Quart Bags.

4. Hunger is my friend, and waiting until I am truly hungry and quitting before I am full are nonnegotiable. Tracking my hunger will expose how I deceive myself.

5. By listing the schemes of Demanding Child in my Ruby Journal and accessing how my Sane Adult really feels, I can dismantle the Demanding Child's tricks, one by one.

6. Failure can be useful, if I will evaluate it and learn from it.

Lesson 7

Finding Substitutes for Self-Soothing and Entertainment

Friday, September 5   *Weight: 167*   *Pounds lost: 8*   *Still to lose: 37*

At five o'clock every day, I could set my watch because Eva enters Zach's office precisely at that time. Usually, she has a joke or story for him. Since she is the self-proclaimed social director at the firm, she makes it her personal responsibility to find out what everybody is doing over the weekend. She even asked me earlier today what I was doing this weekend, and I was happy that I could report that I am not a complete social misfit and that I am actually going to the Train concert tonight.

"What are you and Rachel doing this weekend?" she asks Zach.

"Rachel bought tickets to Train for my birthday last spring, so we're going tonight," he says, emotionless.

Zach and Rachel are going to Train? Immediately I am worried that we will run into them and that they will see that I am getting my dates from the nursing home.

"Oooh," she squeals. "Jackie is going to Train, too. Where are your seats?"

"Not sure, but if I know Rachel, they will be in the center and close to the stage," he says.

Uh, that is where our seats are. Ugh! They will see Gramps again!

"Jackie," Eva calls from Zach's office, "Zach and Rachel are going to Train, too. Where are your seats?"

"I'm not exactly sure," I say, sort of lying and sort of not, because I do not know if they are seats nine and ten or twelve and thirteen—although I do know they are on row nine.

Now, all night long, I will try to hide from Zach and Rachel. What a strain on the night.

Zach walks into my office, hands me some papers to file, and with an expressionless face, says, "Maybe we will run into you tonight," and returns to his office.

It is not a big deal, but I feel embarrassed for Rachel to see how old Brandon is. He is a pretty nice guy and probably the best I can do, but still. She is always a couple notches up on me, and it feels crummy. Rachel and Zach are the Nashville version of Princess Kate and Prince William.

Driving home from work, I notice how horrible Nashville rush-hour traffic is. With that coupled with the dread of the evening, I'm not in good spirits.

"Hello, Young Jackie," a familiar voice says.

Again, I am startled by the sudden appearance of the Genie in my passenger seat. You'd think he could at least make an appointment.

"Today I want to talk about the two—and only two—reasons you eat when you are not hungry," he says. "One reason is for self-soothing, and the second reason is for entertainment. Eating in response to these two situations—instead of only eating in response to true physical hunger—is the major barrier to your success in being thin."

It is preposterous how he tries to take something so complicated and make it ridiculously simple.

"To combat this struggle, you need to do two things," he says. "One, which we have already discussed, is to recognize that Demanding Child is constantly lurking in the shadows, urging you to eat when you are not truly hungry. But number two, which we will discuss today, is to *find alternatives to soothing and entertaining yourself.*"

Nothing else works as quickly as food to soothe me or entertain me.

"I introduced the concept of the Quart Bags earlier," he says. "This is an important strategy to have in place when you simply must eat to dial down emotions but you are not physically hungry. Eventually, I hope you will learn to only eat for true hunger, but the Quart Bags are a helpful strategy to use while you are in the transition of learning to dial down strong emotions. I have noticed that you are still not taking the time to fix your Quart Bags every morning."

"Uh, well, okay, I will do better, Genie." Geesh, I do not appreciate the way this guy creeps on me.

"Also, you can ramp up your selection of herbal teas," he says. "There is a plethora of flavors, such as chocolate, red raspberry, caramel, vanilla, and many more at your grocery store. Simply drinking hot water with lemon can be very relaxing. This strategy has been incredibly helpful to many of my past *Skinny School* students."

Fix the Quart Bags. Buy more herbal tea. Noted.

"Finding other ways to soothe and entertain yourself will be a discovery process," he says. "For example, you will discover many little pleasurable treats, like putting a bathrobe in a dryer for a couple minutes on a chilly winter morning. Having an easily accessible stack of good books to read entertains and soothes many women. Reading magazines, surfing the web, taking hot baths, window shopping, journaling, spending time with a friend, taking a walk at the park, watching TV shows or movies, playing with pets, doing hobbies…the list of where you can find pleasure and comfort is endless."

None of that is as effective as a donut.

"You certainly do not have to give up pleasure or comfort, but you do need to find other pleasure and comfort besides food."

This is a course in itself, trying to find other things that comfort and entertain me. Food has been my best friend, my Prozac, and my stimulation for thirteen years.

"What I am getting ready to tell you could be another whole Genie School in itself, but this principle is so important in overcoming your obsession with food that I must discuss it now. This extremely healing truth *is to find a passion in life*, an overriding goal or interest in which you can immerse and lose yourself. It is imperative, absolutely imperative, that you find something *you are wildly interested in* and devote your thoughts during your free time to a pursuit in which you are gifted and delighted to perform. Part of your obsession with food is that you are not in touch with work that thrills you. Although you are talented in the area of law, you do not feel fulfilled by it. The resources to discover your passion and genius are plentiful, Young Jackie, but honestly, I think you are already in touch with your genius area."

As he says that, I know what he is talking about. Law school is not my passion; writing novels is. And when I immerse myself in fiction writing, I do lose track of time as well as forget about food. I need to think hard about this idea, as my writing is definitely healing for me. Time for working on my novel gets squeezed out, and the Genie is telling me that working on this pursuit would be healing to my crazy eating patterns. Actually, it sounds like he wants me to trade an obsession with food for a focus on something else in which I am wildly interested. Hmmmm…I need to take some time to process that. Maybe my novel writing should be given a higher priority in my life. The mere thought excites me.

"We will now construct List Six in your Ruby Journal, 'Pleasures and Comforts in Life besides Food.' You can list the ideas that we have discussed, as well as add your own to the list as you think of them. In Lesson Twelve, we will discuss dialing down Emotional Tidal Waves. That lesson will give you some further ideas on soothing yourself, too. I am leaving you a new outfit to wear tonight as well as my Genie Broiled Chicken Kebab recipe."

The Genie disintegrates, and it is a good thing because I'm home, and I need to get ready. Although that was a short lesson, I have a feeling it is one that is going to be hugely transformative. Actually, just thinking about giving myself the freedom to work more on my novel is exhilarating. I think I understand how this principle will be healing to my compulsive overeating.

However, as I walk into my apartment, my thoughts are torn away from writing novels because Tory is cooking what looks like a dinner for eight in the kitchen. Recently, she promised to pay me the overdue rent, but I have not approached the subject of her moving out, as I am afraid that if I tell her that, I will never see the past-due rent money.

Seeing Tory cooking in a cute outfit with perfect hair and makeup, I notice a little check in my spirit. Well, maybe she is cooking for a date. I don't know, and I really don't care, as long as she cleans up the dishes.

Instead of dwelling on Tory, I shower and dress for my geriatric date. Brandon might be growing on me by one-half ounce. I mean, the diamond bracelet didn't hurt him.

When he arrives, I meet him at the door, feeling more confident than I have in a while, wearing my new dark jeans and this gold-and-cream top. Being down eight pounds feels good. My new fake diamond earrings dangle down quite a bit and look great with my new bracelet. I have mixed a classy look with just an edge.

Walking to the door, Tory greets Brandon with a loud, overdone, "Hi, Brandon." She engages him in conversation about which cities he has visited this week, and he relates his recent visits to London and Barcelona. Her excitement is again excessive.

I have no jealousy, I don't think, but this repeated idea of Tory hitting on Brandon is annoying. Could she have gone to all that trouble to get dressed up for Brandon? Her spending habits and his checkbook would make a good twosome.

"You two have a good time," she says. "I'm staying home tonight, trying out some new recipes. This international gourmet cooking I'm learning is fascinating."

"What are you making?" Brandon politely asks.

"Coq au vin," she says.

"I had the best coq au vin in Paris last month," he alertly says, raising his energy up a bar. "That is one of my favorite recipes."

Now, as to when Tory started gourmet cooking, I have no idea. It has always been brownies and chocolate-chip cookies before this.

Maybe I am hyper-alert, or maybe I am being over suspicious, but something is amiss here. The gourmet cooking, the teased hair and makeup, the overfriendliness to Brandon…something smells wrong, and my judgmental nature tells me that my roommate is after my date with the big bank account. However, Brandon is only mildly friendly and focuses on me. "Ready to go?" he asks.

He is dressed in expensive blue jeans, ones that have too much design on the rear pockets for an old geezer. Those jeans are reserved for those of us under thirty. He has on a nice starched long-sleeve navy shirt that is tucked in. Even though he is forty-eight, his waistline is that of a younger man, so two more points for Brandon.

Chatting in his car about his travel and business, I realize again that Brandon is very nice. "Tell me about your first two weeks at your new job," he says. "What surprised you that you were not expecting?"

Leaving out all the drama with Eva, I only talk about the cases and the work. Brandon asks very good questions, and I enjoy talking about myself with someone attentively listening. He is up another one-half ounce. I try not to look at the wrinkles around his eyes.

Arriving at the concert, Brandon and I move slowly with the large crowd, all of whom are also trying to find their seats. There is an electric feel to a crowd who is out on Friday night, free from the week's work grind and ready to enjoy some great music. Feeling the energy of the crowd, my energy is pulled up, too. But my energy drops when I look at Brandon, and I notice his shoes. He has on business dress shoes with jeans, like my dad would wear. Not really sure why, but it bothers me. Maybe I can get over the age difference—but then, maybe not.

Walking down to the ninth row, I keep my antennas up for Zach and Rachel. So far, so good. But not for long. As we approach the seats, I see they are seated four rows directly behind our seats. Brandon and I will be in their direct view all night. My stomach begins to churn as I realize that Rachel and Zach will be looking at my derriere as well as my decrepit date all night long.

Trying to act like I don't see them, I walk down the aisle. Brandon catches Zach's eye and waves. "Isn't that your boss that we saw at the restaurant?" he asks. Of course it is, but I act surprised. Smiling sweetly, I wave at Zach. Rachel is on her phone and doesn't see us—or at least, she acts like she doesn't.

The warm-up band begins, and Brandon claps along to a song he knows. What is it about how old people clap and how young people clap that is different? Brandon's old-person clapping annoys me again. I am not sure how or why. Is it how he shakes his hips while he claps? Or how he rocks back and forth? I am way too picky, I realize, to get irritated over how someone claps, but anyhow, I do. I look at my pretty bracelet from Dubai and decide his clapping is okay.

Before Train begins, I tell Brandon that I am going to the restroom. Leaving the seats, I walk up toward the landing.

"Jackie," I hear a familiar voice say from behind me. It is Zach, and Rachel is not with him. Surely she found one of her high-bred friends and is gabbing with them.

"Hey, Zach," I say. He is trying to get to me, politely stepping around people. I wait for him to get to where I am.

"How is your night going?" he asks.

"I guess okay," I say. Something about Zach makes me feel like I have been given a truth serum. I don't know why, but I start babbling. "This is the second time I have been out with Brandon and…I don't know, but he seems a little old, and it keeps bothering me," I say. Now I am embarrassed. I mean, he was just asking "How is your night going?" like one would ask, "How is the weather?" But stupid me—I have to go and get all honest and tell him how I feel. It is hard being me.

"Brandon seems like a really nice guy to me," he says. "But if the age bothers you, that is important. You will soon know if this is a dead end." Zach slightly smiles.

I light up. What is it about when someone gets you and says something that connects? I mean, Zach understands. I am not dating like I was in high school—just so I will have a date for a dance. At twenty-eight, one dates to find a possible marriage partner.

Leaving Zach and walking toward the ladies' restroom, I experience that familiar contentment I get after even a brief encounter with Zach. Why does he always have to understand?

The awareness of Zach and Rachel's presence haunts me the entire night. Train is amazing, and when the concert is over, I take a ridiculous amount of time after the encore to gather my things—hoping that Zach and Rachel will be far gone, and we will not have to run into them. Nevertheless, they are waiting for us at the top of the landing. Rachel has her hands wrapped around Zach's arms, as to signify to the world what is her rightful property.

We all discuss how terrific the concert was, while I secretly survey Rachel's outfit. Skinny jeans from Anthropologie, probably a size zero. A beige, cotton, woven top with insets of paisley patches. Classy, adorable. She is stylish, skinny, and I hate it. The feeling that I had earlier that I looked nice tonight is completely gone, and I feel like Big Bird on *Sesame Street*.

"Do you guys want to join us and get something to eat?" Zach says to Brandon, ignoring me. I watch Rachel as she squeezes Zach's arm, as if to signal something. Obviously, she is signaling him to stop, to not ask the help to meet them for dinner.

"Thank you, Zach," Brandon begins, "but I have been out of the country two weeks, and Jackie and I need to catch up." It is embarrassing the way he says it, like we have got some connection and we need to reignite it. But what can I say? And I certainly do not want to go anywhere with snotty Rachel. Rachel looks relieved and loosens her grip on Zach's arm.

"Maybe another time," Zach says, and we all depart in different directions. Simmering, I feel upset that Rachel views me as either the help or as the fat girl from high school. Either way, it feels uncomfortable. And then, I do not like the way Brandon portrayed us as needing to reconnect, like we are a couple. That old familiar anxiety of being upset and not knowing what to do with it appears again.

Right before Zach and Rachel get out of earshot, she turns to me and asks, "Jackie, are you taking Brandon to the wedding in two weeks?" Sick that she brought it up, and feeling that it was entirely out of place for her to do so, I now feel like I have to invite him. Maybe he will be out of the country.

"Not yet," I say. Shouldn't Rachel know better than to ask those questions at her age?

Zach's eyes find mine and hold. I am sure it is only a gesture on his part to be a good friend, to communicate that he knows Rachel should not ask those questions, but the chemical explosion from the eye lock for me is insane.

When Zach and Rachel walk off, I feel obliged to ask Brandon to the wedding. Please, please be out of town. "Attorney Simpson's son is getting married two weeks from tomorrow. Would you like to go?" I do not know why I am so hard on Brandon. He is nice, educated, and loaded. Really, he would be terribly attractive if I was entering menopause.

"I would love to go and meet everyone you work with. Thank you for inviting me," he says, as he grabs my hand as we walk toward the car.

Brandon and I get to the car, and he sings a little "Hey, Soul Sister" that we just heard Train sing. Sorry, but again, it grosses me out. I have got to get over being turned off by his innocent behaviors. He is such a nice guy, and he acts like he really likes me. Maybe he will grow on me.

And then again, maybe not.

The nonnegotiables in *Skinny School* so fa-r are:

1. I expect to work like a Champion to retrain my mind since this is a current Top Four Life Goal.
2. Ditching sweets and starches is not optional if I want to overhaul my metabolism. I am to track my sugar/carb grams as well as my calories. I focus on all the beautiful, delicious food *I get to eat* instead of what I must not eat.
3. Planning and prepping are the secrets Champions use to conquer goals. I must daily make Quart Bags.
4. Hunger is my friend, and waiting until I am truly hungry and quitting before I am full are nonnegotiable. Tracking my hunger is imperative and will expose how I deceive myself with wanting to eat for self-soothing and entertainment.
5. By listing the schemes of Demanding Child in my Ruby Journal and accessing how my Sane Adult really feels, I can dismantle the Demanding Child's tricks, one by one.
6. Failure can be useful, if I will evaluate it and learn from it.
7. Finding substitutes for soothing and entertaining myself besides using food is crucial. Discovering my passion and immersing myself in it will be extremely healing to my food obsession.

Lesson 8

Insist on a Clean Environment

Thursday, September 11 Weight: 165   Pounds lost: 10   Still to lose: 35

After getting all the demand packages out, finishing another draft on one of Zach's briefs, and returning all the phone calls, I am through with all my work. I like that about me—efficient, capable, kind of a can-do girl. Walking into Zach's office, I ask if he has anything else I can do to help him.

I love that look on his face, the astonished look of "Wow, you are kidding, right?"

"Jackie, I think I will take the afternoon off, go play golf, and let you run my law practice," he says. He is not thinking about playing golf. He is telling me how valuable I am, how helpful I am to him, how capable I am.

"Should I call and get you a tee time?" I ask.

He does that adorable thing when the grin tries to appear, but he represses it.

"Maybe next week," he says, but we both know that Zach would never play golf during the workday.

It is lunchtime, so I walk to my car to run a few errands. The starter in my car has gone out. After calling a tow truck service, I call Beth to see if she can pick me up from work. The answer is, of course, yes.

At quitting time when I get in Beth's car, she asks, "Why don't we run by your apartment, get some jeans, and then you come home with me to have dinner with us? Richard is working out at the gym, so we can chat and cook dinner together while we wait on him. Then I will run you home after dinner."

Since I was not a Champion today, and I have not planned my dinner, I am very happy to accept the offer. Beth is fun no matter what we are doing, and not eating scrambled eggs alone sounds great.

At my apartment, I grab my favorite pair of jeans, an oversized yellow shirt, and some flip-flops. My feet would really like my UGG house shoes, but still, I decide against being that comfy.

Arriving at Beth's house, I immediately feel at home. Her cream-and-gold decorating is elegant, with modern clean lines. We begin cleaning and chopping mushrooms, onions, garlic, and parsley. Just looking at the healthy food makes me happy that I'm treating my body well. And I'm glad I'm not alone tonight. Being single kind of stinks.

"Oh, no, I'm out of parmesan cheese," Beth says. "I can't make Alfredo sauce for the shrimp without Parmesan cheese!"

"Want me to run to the store?" I ask.

"Oh, would you, Jackie? That would be great." I start to get my purse to leave, and Beth's cell phone rings. I can tell it is her husband, Richard, by the way she talks to him.

"Yes, really, that would be fine," she says. "I have enough. I already invited Jackie and she is here, so that would be fun."

Beth listens some more and adds, "Sure. He can shower in the guest bathroom…Love you, too."

My heart starts to fall to my stomach. I know that Richard works out with Zach, and the thought that Zach might be coming to dinner throws my equilibrium. But they would not invite Zach over without Rachel. It must be someone else.

"That was Richard," she says. "Rachel is at some college sorority reunion tonight and Zach is free, so Richard invited Zach over to eat with us, too."

As nonchalantly as I can, I say, "Oh, that is nice." But on the inside, I am anything but nonchalant. I start thinking about how I look—about my hair, about my clothes, about my makeup. Oh, why did I not wear that pink shirt that just came back from the cleaners? And thank goodness I did not wear my UGG house shoes!

"Where are your keys, Beth? I better get going so I can get that Parmesan cheese." I feel kind of panicky now that Zach is coming.

Beth starts digging through her purse, looking for her keys. As she hunts for them, she starts talking. "Now I am not supposed to tell this, and I want you to promise not to tell," Beth begins. I make a mental note to remember not to tell Beth something if I care that it doesn't get told.

"Okay, sure," I say, thinking about how I need to freshen up my makeup before the guys get here. Maybe I can do that in the car.

"Zach told Richard that Mr. Hanover, Rachel's dad, called him and said that since Zach and Rachel had been dating two years, he wanted Zach to know there was a two-carat ring in the family that Zach could give to Rachel when he was ready," Beth said, her eyes as round as the cherry tomatoes I was just slicing.

"Rachel's dad called Zach?" I ask, hardly believing the story.

"Yes, this week," Beth says. "I guess with Christmas coming, the Hanovers are expecting an engagement, and so Rachel's dad called him to offer the ring."

"Maybe Zach and Rachel have already discussed their engagement, and so her dad felt comfortable calling him," I say, still worried about how washed out I must look and wondering if I brought my makeup.

"Zach told Richard he has never even mentioned engagement to Rachel," Beth says. "This is all Mr. Hanover's idea. It was inappropriate, if you ask me," Beth continues.

I guess Zach wants to surprise Rachel, I think to myself. That is why they have not discussed it. But I agree with Beth that the boldness of Mr. Hanover was over the line. But maybe the family feels close enough to Zach to discuss engagement.

"I will be back in a minute, Beth," I say, grabbing her keys and heading out the door. This conversation is very interesting, but I cannot look like this when Zach comes in, whether he is getting engaged soon or not.

As soon as I get in Beth's car, I open my purse to see if I brought my makeup. Dang, I did not!

"I thought you might need this," says the passenger who appears to my right. **The Genie is sitting there, holding my makeup bag.** I cannot help but grin.

"Our time together is limited tonight, I realize," he begins, "but I want to quickly discuss the benefit of keeping a Clean Environment in your kitchen."

I'm not a perfect housekeeper by any means, but I certainly keep things tidy. Why is he talking about a clean kitchen?

"The term *Clean Environment* refers to *not having Trash Food in your kitchen*. Young Jackie, do you know that you can predict if a youth will do drugs by knowing *how often* drugs are offered to him? You are weak humans, and you often succumb to temptation in proportion to how often something is offered to you. That is why many wise married men do not have attractive secretaries, as the continual temptation makes saying no more difficult. Humans are very limited beings, and they only have so many Willpower Points to resist temptation. Wise humans guard the areas where they know they are easily tempted."

So where exactly is he going with this?

"If you have a kitchen and pantry that are stashed with alluring Trash Food, you are setting yourself up for failure," he says. "Do not buy Trash Food, and if someone gives you some, give it away or throw it away. Keep a Clean Environment, one free of tempting Trash Food."

Beth struggles with her weight, too. Although she loves to cook with organic ingredients, I saw the contents of her pantry: cereals, cookies, crackers, and much more. To be honest, some of that food is still in my pantry, too.

"Women say they have to keep Trash Food around for their kids or for company, but with some planning and savviness, women can wean their kids off Trash Food. Many women keep deviled eggs, deli meats, fruits, and scrumptious leftovers in the fridge, and the kids are thrilled. You do not have to keep Trash Food around."

My sister Jessica would disagree. Her pantry is full of Trash Food for her boys.

"This is a short lesson, but temptation that is easily accessible is hard to withstand. Your limited daily Willpower Points will not be spent saying no to Trash Food items if they are not there to begin with. Fill your fridge and pantry with all the fabulous food we have discussed for the past month, and feel happy that you have the discipline and willpower to not bring Trash Food into your kitchen."

I understand why ex-smokers should stay away from people who smoke, and I understand that people who have drinking problems should stay away from situations where there is alcohol. But I never thought about trying to stay away from Trash Food. It is as if Trash Food has a rightful and dutiful place in our lives. Fortunately, I am learning the error of that thought. Trash Food should be disposed of...or at the very least, quarantined.

"I left some Genie Spinach Salad with Goat Cheese and Bacon with Caesar Dressing in your refrigerator for tomorrow," he says and disappears, just as I pull into the grocery store parking lot. I hurry in, get the Parmesan cheese, rush back to the car, apply some makeup, and then quickly return to Beth's house.

Walking back into the kitchen, I notice that Beth has turned off the overhead lights and has lit candles. The room has a warm glow, and the smell of the mushrooms sautéing in the wine is alluring. Beth looks at me and then does a double-take. The knowing look on her face says it all. The light bulb just went on for Beth. A woman shows her heart when she fixes her hair and makeup.

In the softest and sweetest of voices, Beth says, "Jackie, you look very pretty." I am not sure why, but her comment makes me want to cry. Then I realize it is because that is exactly how my mom, who died four years ago in a car wreck, used to talk to me. She would stare at me, and in a soft voice say, with the most sincere heart, "Jackie, you look pretty." Mom loved me more than she loved herself. And although she knew I was sad that I struggled with forty-five extra pounds, she always found ways to tell me how bright I was, how witty I was, or how pretty I was. Hearing Beth say the words that my mother used to say, and in the same tone, makes me ache to see my mom. I have not told anyone about my crush on my boss, but I could have told my mom. I could have told her how I know he is out of my league but that he excites me every time he smiles and tells me how much I help him. She would not beat me up for having a crush on him, even though he has a girlfriend. She would have told me that *he* was missing out. I miss her badly right now. When my mom was killed in that car wreck, I lost my best friend and my encourager. My sister Jessica has tried to replace Mom and be there for me, but it is not the same.

"Can you get the glasses out of the cabinet and fill them with water, please?" Beth asks me. I forget I am supposed to be helping prepare dinner. Guys like Zach Boltz do that to girls.

Men's voices appear at the front door. Zach and Richard walk in, laughing over something. They are both in their sweaty gym clothes. Zach does not spend much money on clothes. He is wearing a pair of gym shorts that he probably had in college with a T-shirt from a mission trip he took five years ago. I notice clothes, and Zach wears the same four suits to work over and over again, mixing up his look with different shirts and ties. Fashion is not something Zach puts a high price on, even though he looks very nice and professional every day.

Suddenly, I am embarrassed. The soft music, the candles! Why, this all looks like Beth and I set up this romantic evening so Zach would be with me. Oh, my gosh! Surely he would not think that, would he? I feel terrible. I have to let Zach know I had no part of this. I have to.

"Hi, Jackie," Zach says.

"Hi," I say. Dang, I hate how tongue-tied I get around him. If this was the president of the United States, I could think of something clever to say, but I freeze around Zach.

"I bet you guys are probably sick of each other after working together all week, but try to be nice to each other," Richard says. He is trying to be funny and lighten up the moment, but it does not work at all.

"Not me," Zach says, the good-natured person he is. "Jackie is always fun to have around." And he tosses me one of his Ralph-Lauren-on-the-sailboat grins. Thank goodness no one else knows when my stomach flips.

"I got invited at the last minute, too," I say, wanting him to know that this was not a premeditated fix-up.

I do not know if he understood what I was saying or not, but thankfully, he is wise enough to change the subject. "Something smells good, Beth," he says, and she launches into all the fresh, organic ingredients she is using tonight. Zach tries to act interested.

The guys shower, and Beth and I finish preparing dinner. Beth and Richard are drinking wine with their dinner, but Zach and I both do not drink, so we are having water with lemon. Looking at Zach across the candlelit table makes me feel a little drunk, though.

I am anything but relaxed. I am still worried Zach might think this is a setup.

At first, the guys do most of the talking, about sports, about the gym. Halfway through dinner, Richard blurts out (maybe it was the wine), "By the way, my parents are not using their four season tickets to the Titans next weekend, and we four can use them."

Immediately we are all silent, and Richard realizes what a mistake he made with that comment. Why, of course, Zach would need to bring Rachel, and now Richard feels bad he said that in front of me. Richard usually does not make faux pas like that, but the truth is that Beth and Richard do not love Rachel either.

The table is ridiculously quiet, and I feel compelled to break the tension. "My sister Jessica will be here next weekend to visit, but maybe I can go another time." She is actually only driving through Nashville and stopping for lunch. I know I stretched the truth a little. I never claimed to be perfect.

That comment seems to work to rebound the conversation to its prior light-hearted banter. Back to sports, music, movies, books...we jump from topic to topic, all four of us having different opinions. We laugh, we talk, we tease. Zach is currently reading *To Kill a Mockingbird* for the third time. He is telling us about one of his favorite scenes, when Boo Radley saves Atticus's kids. Beth and Richard have not read the book, but I have.

"Zach, of course you like that book," I say. "You are the modern day Atticus Finch."

Beth asks, "What does that mean? Who is Atticus Finch, and why is Zach like him?"

But Zach knows what I mean, and his eyes rise to meet mine. Atticus Finch is the protagonist, who is also a lawyer. He is kind, stable, unselfish, and willing to put himself in harm's way to help others. The compliment is sincere, and Zach hears it.

Before I can answer Beth's questions, her sister calls and she takes it, although she tells her sister she will call her back later. Beth then forgets about her question, and I let it drop, too.

We all four decide we will tell about a scene in a movie that we have enjoyed. Richard tells a funny Jim Carrey scene in *Dumb and Dumber.* Beth describes a scene with Meg Ryan in *You've Got Mail.* Zach describes a courtroom scene in *A Few Good Men,* and now it is my turn.

"I like a scene in *Rear Window* with Jimmy Stewart and Grace Kelly," I say. "Jimmy Stewart does not think Grace Kelly's high breeding would work with his life since he is a world-traveling photographer. He is going to break up with her because she is too refined and could not understand the 'combat boot' part of his job. But later in the movie, when the two of them are trying to solve a murder, Grace Kelly is climbing up lattices and sneaking through windows in daring ways to help solve the murder. He is surprised by how brave and adventurous his girlfriend truly is."

Richard and Beth's baby, Alexis, is crying, and they both get up to see what the matter is. Zach and I are left alone at the table. "Are you like that, Jackie? Would we all be surprised by who you are on the inside?"

The question rocks me. We were just sharing favorite movie scenes. Where did this come from? What is he asking?

I do not answer because I cannot think of anything to say.

"I can see you climbing lattices and jumping on board to help solve a murder," he says. "Is that why you like that scene? Because of the adventure? Or because you like to use your brain to think and figure things out?"

Not having really analyzed before why I love this scene, I answer without thinking through my answer. "What I love about the scene is that Jimmy

Stewart thought he knew his girlfriend, and he was judging her on how she dressed and presented herself. He had missed her heart altogether."

"Do you think you like that scene because maybe other people do not get the real you?" he asks.

Startled again by this question and feeling uncovered and unmasked, I quickly realize that is exactly the reason I love that scene.

Before I can respond to that question, Beth and Richard return. The four of us continue our banter. I talk, Beth talks, Richard talks, Zach talks. We all laugh and talk some more. Everyone contributes. But Zach especially laughs at everything I say. At one point while laughing, he asks, "Jackie, who writes your material?"

It is 9:30 p.m., and I remember tomorrow is a workday. I blew off my LSAT studying tonight (which I am thinking about giving up, anyhow, after that session with the Genie on finding your passion), and I also neglected to do my grocery shopping. Now I am worried about what I am going to pack for lunch tomorrow. Well, this was worth it. I loved tonight. Absolutely, positively adored tonight. Maybe I can get up early and run to the grocery.

"Beth, let's clean up these dishes and then maybe you can take me home," I say.

"Where is your car?" Zach asks.

"In the shop. The starter went out," I say.

"I will take you home," he offers. "You are on my way home."

Beth does not miss a beat. "That would help me so much, Zach," she says. "You two go on. I know it is late. These dishes will just take a second, and Richard will help me."

"I am going to bed," Richard teases. "They are all yours, Beth." But we know better than to believe him.

There is really no way to argue after what Beth says, so I get my purse, and Zach and I head to his car. The evening is cool and crisp. The crickets and other insects are so loud that you almost think it is animated sound, coming piped in through some speakers.

Settling into his front passenger seat, I realize that I have never been in such a small, confined space with Zach in the dark. The chemistry I feel for him is crazy, energy that is strong and pulsating. We drive a little and do not talk. Feeling uncomfortable with the silence, I have to break it.

"Richard and Beth are certainly great friends," I say. A stupid thing to say, but I could not think of anything better.

"*Great* friends," he repeats. "I thoroughly enjoyed the evening."

He does not look at me, but I glance at his profile with the help of the streetlights. His perfect, masculine profile.

"How do you like working at Simpson Law so far, Jackie?" I am not sure why he is asking me this. Probably because he is trying to come up with conversation, just like I am.

"I like it a lot," I honestly say. "You are easy to work for. I like listening to how you handle your clients. I have never seen a lawyer handle clients with the compassion and genuineness that you do. It has changed how I feel about how lawyers should practice law."

He looks at me to read my expression, and I can tell that my remark means a lot to him. "Thanks, Jackie. That is nice to hear."

"It's true," I say. "I hear you giving people advice all the time that won't benefit you, but just to help them. That is how all lawyers should act."

Again, the pleasure covers his face, and he glances at me with a grin. He just looks and doesn't say anything, which makes me nervous and uncomfortable.

"I enjoy having you work for me, more than you know," he says. "I have never had competent help like you before."

My heart sinks as he says this, as I realize again, for the billionth time, that for Zach this is professional, and for me it is personal. I am mad at myself for the way I keep thinking that Zach has more than a professional friendship and respect for me. Dang it, Jackie! I say to myself. He has a gorgeous girlfriend who is probably getting a two-carat family ring for Christmas. Quit it! Give up this thing you have for Zach.

"And you are a great friend, Jackie. I really enjoy your company. No one makes me laugh more than you. Richard was talking earlier about having a guys' night out, and he asked me to think of some guys to invite who would be fun. I thought of you," he says, as if that was a great compliment.

I am not sure what to do with that comment. The Rachels of the world date the great guys, and I am merely the friend of the great guys. I feel like crying, but I know that I have to keep it together for another two to three minutes until I am out of the car. I am not thinking about what I am saying really; I am just trying to make conversation until I can get home. "My grandfather used to call me Jack, because he said I was like one of the boys." The tears are begging to roll, but I keep the dam from breaking.

Zach glances at me, and our eyes briefly meet.

"I like that name, Jack. That is what I am going to call you. It fits you," he says as he again glances at the hippopotamus in his passenger seat. I am a funny, witty, smart, buddy-like hippopotamus. This is so typical of my life.

"Jack—what a great name for you," he repeats, as we pull up to my apartment. I thank him and tell him I will see him in the morning. As I get out of the car, the dam breaks. I do not turn around because I don't want him to see the waterworks. I open the door to my apartment, walk straight to my bed, and sob for a good ten minutes. Maybe fifteen. Yup, good ole funny, fat Jack. That is certainly me.

The pull of the refrigerator to medicate my despair is strong, but I grab my Quart Bags, gulping down some celery and cherry tomatoes.

When I lose this blasted weight, I will find my own Prince Charming. There are other Zach Boltzs out there, I tell myself.

But I have a hard time fooling myself. There are not any other Zach Boltzs anywhere on the planet. And this one is getting ready to get engaged.

The nonnegotiables in *Skinny School* so far are:

1. I expect to work like a Champion to retrain my mind since this is a Top Four Life Goal.
2. Ditching sweets and starches is not optional if I want to overhaul my metabolism. I am to track my sugar/carb grams as well as my calories. I focus on all the beautiful, delicious food *I get to eat* instead of what I must not eat.

3. Planning and prepping are the secrets Champions use to conquer goals. I must daily make Quart Bags.
4. Hunger is my friend, and waiting until I am truly hungry and quitting before I am full are nonnegotiable. Tracking my hunger is imperative and will expose how I deceive myself with wanting to eat for self-soothing and entertainment.
5. By listing the schemes of Demanding Child in my Ruby Journal and accessing how my Sane Adult really feels, I can dismantle the Demanding Child's tricks, one by one.
6. Failure can be useful, if I will evaluate it and learn from it.
7. Finding substitutes for soothing and entertaining myself besides using food is imperative. Discovering my passion and immersing myself in it will be extremely healing to my food obsession.
8. A clean environment, one without Trash Food, is crucial to reduce temptation.

Lesson 9

Make Appointments with Yourself to Exercise

Saturday, September 20 Weight: 161   Pounds lost: 14   Still to lose: 31

Gramps and I are on our way to Attorney Simpson's son's wedding. I have been ridiculously nervous about everyone seeing my nursing home escort. At least Brandon knows how to dress well. His blue pinstripe suit looks like something an Arab prince or a corporate tycoon would wear, probably a Gucci or an Yves Saint Laurent. It is a far cry from my dress from T. J. Maxx for $24.99. Again, Brandon showed up with an extravagant gift, some David Yurman earrings from London. Really, I feel guilty accepting his extravagant gifts, but I don't know what else to do.

Being fourteen pounds lighter does make me feel more confident than I have in a while. Plus this goldish-colored dress is mega slenderizing. I wonder what Ravishing Rachel will have on.

Eva is in the wedding, of course, and truly looks like a Barbie doll. The soft blue dresses of the bridesmaids are beautiful, and Eva is so pretty that she shows up the bride. I think she knows it, too. Brandon and I sit an appropriate ten rows back, and Zach and Rachel sit two rows in front of us. Zach has on his darkest charcoal suit with a starched white shirt and my favorite yellow tie. He is to die for. His future wife is wearing a spaghetti-strapped black dress with pearls embroidered on the front. Classy, of course. Understated and elegant. Just looking at her upper-class refinement makes me feel frumpy.

During the minister's sermon, Brandon grabs my hand. His hands look like my dad's hands, and I am once again—grossed out.

At the end of the ceremony, Rachel leans over and whispers into Zach's ear. She is probably telling him that she does not want the flowers in their wedding to look like these, or maybe she is whispering about the music they should have in their wedding. Nestling up under his shoulder, she looks like she is the soon-to-be wife. Zach does not lean toward her or put his arm around her, though. Typical buttoned-up Zach.

After the ceremony, Brandon and I move to the reception area, and Eva is already there with champagne in her hand and her shoes off, ready to party hardy. The band is playing, and Eva begins the dancing with her arms over her head in wild abandon.

Brandon goes to the men's room, and I hear a voice behind me say, "Are you having a good time?"

Recognizing the voice, I catch my breath. It is Zach. I don't know where Rachel is and neither do I care.

"Not bad," I say. As I'm trying to think of something witty to say, the usual brain freeze hits me.

"You look nice in that dress, Jackie." I look at Zach's sincere face and know he means it. He is not flirting. He is simply being friendly.

"Thank you," I say, tongue-tied. Again, I can do nothing but flash him my best smile. My heart rate is sky-high and I hate that he has this power over me.

We both causally chitchat about the wedding as we watch Eva seriously compete with J. Lo as far as who is the best dancer.

"Does Brandon like to dance?" Zach asks.

"I do not know," I say, "I guess I will find out tonight. Does Rachel?"

"Rachel rates dancing up there with shopping," he says, stone faced at first, but that gives in to one of his boyish grins. I laugh, as I know what he is saying. We both know how much time and money Rachel spends shopping.

Brandon approaches us as the band starts playing Earth, Wind, and Fire's "Boogie Wonderland."

"Aw, this is a favorite song," Brandon says. "Hi, Zach. Come on, Jackie, let's dance." He grabs my hand and pulls me toward the dance floor. Brandon was in his twenties when this song first came out and I...I was not born.

As I leave Zach, I catch his eye. There is that eye contact again, that eye lock. I know it is just professional friends for him, but for me, it feels like zest and color and stimulation and life. Zach's eyes make me want to push PAUSE and never resume play.

Leaving those thoughts, Brandon begins to tear up the dance floor. I mean, he is almost like a professional, he is so good. Wow, Gramps can dance. Noticing Zach shuffling around on the dance floor with Rachel, I realize dancing is not Zach's strong suit.

Time for a slow song. Really, I would rather get some more iced tea, but Brandon wants to dance. Okay, okay, I will. I mean, I *am* his date. His arms get tighter around me. Why does this bother me so much? "This feels nice, babe. Real nice," he says.

I do not think I can take this anymore. I am grossed out to the max. It feels like I have a date with Mr. Rogers of Mr. Rogers' Neighborhood.

Finally, the song is over, and Zach is waiting on the edge of the dance floor. "Jack, bring Justin Timberlake over here and come sit with us."

Rachel is not going to like fat, unpopular high school me sitting at her uppity table, but too bad—her future husband invited us.

Zach directs me to sit by him. Rachel gives me a quick, "Hi, Jackie," and then gets up to tell somebody something that is obviously hilarious. Maybe the old banana split joke.

Soon, though, Rachel is back, pulling on Zach's arm. "Excuse me," he says to Brandon and me, "Rachel wants me to go look at the bride and groom cakes. As you might guess, bridal cakes are in my top three areas of interest in life."

Zach's deadpan look makes me smile. Zach always directs his wit to me, knowing that I am an audience who will predictably appreciate his humor.

I watch them walk off, Cleopatra and Mark Antony. Gorgeous. Of course they are looking at cakes. That is what you do when you are getting ready to get engaged. Of course they are going to be Mr. and Mrs. Zach Boltz, and she will have a Vera Wang wedding dress in a size zero. And of course there will soon be little Zachites running all over the place in smocked outfits with knee socks and saddle oxfords. And the little girls will have bows half the size of their entire heads. They will say "Yes, ma'am" and "No, ma'am" at three years old. It is coming sooner rather than later, so why do I let myself obsess over Zach? At least no one knows. Not Beth. Not Jessica. No one.

Brandon is telling me a story about a restaurant in Dubai, and I can hardly listen, keeping one eye on Zach and Rachel. They are returning to the table. In front of everyone at the table, Zach says, "I know that women carry on about dresses, cakes, flowers, and photography at weddings. However, there is only one thing that is important at a wedding...and that is how good the food is for the guests." Rachel sort of hits him, like she owns him and he should quit teasing.

Brandon says, "Hear, hear!" and offers his glass to Zach to toast. Again, the comment grosses me out.

"Brandon," I whisper, "are you ready to leave?" I am ready to get out of here. I am ready to tell Brandon we cannot date anymore. I cannot take it anymore when he grabs my hand or puts his hand on top of mine. The thought of kissing him is making me want to gag.

Riding back to my apartment, Brandon begins tapping on the steering wheel, singing another Earth, Wind, and Fire song, "Got to Get You into My Life." Not surprisingly, it grosses me out again. Bon Jovi or no Bon Jovi, earrings or no earrings, I cannot keep this up. When we pull up to my apartment, I am ready to give my speech and get out of the car. But before I start, he asks me if he can use my restroom. What can I say? I have to let him.

He comes in and Tory is there. Tory slips away and comes back in a moment with makeup on and her hair foophed up. Tory and Brandon chat and laugh. I can hardly take it. I tell him I have to get up early, and we walk to his car. He begins to move forward like he is coming in for a kiss. I want to say, "In your next life, buddy."

Well, I hate to crush him, but here goes: "Brandon, I think you are a real nice guy, but I don't think we should go out anymore. I hope you can find someone else to take to Bon Jovi." There. I said it. I hope he is not broken, in despair, completely demolished.

"Could you please text me Tory's contact info?" he quickly asks. "Maybe she could go."

"Tory?" I ask. "As in, my roommate?" I do not know why I am so surprised. She has been hitting on him since the day she met him. And he is not upset at all but sort of excited about the hope of Tory going.

"Sure," I say. "I will text you her contact info right now." I send him the info, and he drives off.

Walking inside, I hear Tory talking on the phone in her room. "Bon Jovi? I would *love* to go! Oh, I am so excited, Brandon," and gush, gush, gush.

Again, I am thrilled to be rid of Brandon, but at the same time, I'm a little insulted at how this love affair has been brewing under my nose. I can hear Tory's high, shrill giggles from my room. **And then, as if I have not had enough drama for the night, the Genie appears.**

"Tonight we are going to discuss a topic that makes most women wince," he begins.

As if I have already not had enough wincing for the night.

"The importance of this topic goes beyond weight loss," he says. "In fact, even if this topic did not help with weight loss, you should still perform it for the other health benefits. However, this topic is very important in weight loss, and the topic is exercise," he says.

Oh, no. Exercise? I knew this was eventually coming. Rat tails and hogwash.

"Young Jackie, what if you heard about a new pill that reverses aging, reduces anxiety, increases longevity, decreases blood pressure, releases human growth hormone for youthfulness, steam lines the body for sleekness and youthful appearance, releases endorphins that elevate one's mood, and unclogs metabolism, thereby changing hormones from a fat-storing mode into a fat-burning mode? What if it also decreased PMS symptoms, created healthier body image, improved memory, improved self-confidence, and inspired creativity? Would you be interested in that pill?"

"I would pop two," I answer, "and then relax with the Food Network."

He smiles. "That list I just gave you is only a small portion of the benefits of exercise. You cannot afford not to exercise if you are responsibly taking care of the one body you have been given to last your entire lifetime," he says.

I hate it when he lays this guilt on me, making me responsible for my choices.

"Knowing that exercise is nonnegotiable and crucial to your health is the first point I wanted to discuss tonight," he says.

Somewhere in my subconscious, I knew that. You would have to live in the desert without any media to not have heard of the benefits of exercise. But still. I have been able to push the need to exercise out of my mind. Until, of course, now.

"The second point I would like to make tonight is the necessity of putting exercise in your day as an *appointment*," he continues. "Exercise will not happen unless you make an appointment with yourself. Is morning, noon, or evening a better time for you?"

"I am stiff in the morning, Genie, and I like to sleep in. I don't want to get sweaty at noon and then go back to work, and I'm tired at night. Is there a fourth option?"

His soft face tells me that he is not angry with me for my excuses. But if I know the Genie, I am not going to get by with this. He doesn't speak, but waits.

"Well," I stammer, "I guess the best option would be to get up early and get it over. But then I would have to go to bed earlier, since my sleep is very important to me."

"That is excellent thinking!" he says. "These are the kind of decisions that women do not make by accident. Women must seriously wrestle with the necessity of finding the time to exercise and then devising strategy so it will happen."

I do waste time at night surfing the web, so I guess I could try going to bed earlier.

"You do not *find* the time, you *make* the time, because this is one of your current Top Four Life Goals," he says. "Being healthy necessitates exercising. The only bad workout is the one that did not happen."

I have had a lot of those.

"If you have time to be on Facebook, you have time to exercise," he says.

Whoa...I am not giving up Facebook.

"The next decision you must make is *what specific exercise you will choose to do*," he says. "I have worked with many women, trying to help them uncover the answer to this question, and I have found that there is no single answer. Women must discover what they will actually *do*. In other words, swimming may sound like a great idea, but the logistics of finding a pool, getting wet, etcetera, may actually make swimming a bad choice."

Lying in bed with my laptop and a snack is a good choice.

"I have included two new pages in your Ruby Journal. List Seven is called 'Benefits of Exercise,' and List Eight is called 'What Exercise Will I Do?' I have started filling out the first page. Let's write down some examples on the second page, What Exercise Will I Do?"

"Genie, I like ballroom dancing," I say, thinking of how fun it was to dance tonight, even though my partner was about as sexy as Shrek.

"Yes, ballroom dancing is a good exercise," he says. "But is it realistic that you will find a partner and dance five times a week? Ballroom dancing is probably not going to work for a day-in-day-out exercise program."

Bummer. Okay, I will suggest something else. "I like horseback riding," I say, thinking about when I was a child at summer camp.

"Again, that is a great exercise," he says. "But do you have a horse nearby that you can consistently ride?"

Everything I say, he disses.

"Those exercises are great if they are available for you to regularly do," he says. "However, I think we need to keep thinking. You need to find something that you will do consistently."

Being especially tired tonight after the drama of the wedding and Brandon, I feel he should bring up this difficult subject when I feel better. Like, in a year or two.

"For example, maybe you want to try walking as it is easily available," he continues. "Maybe you could walk with a friend and, at the same time, have a good airing of your soul. Or maybe you could walk with your phone and music. This is an exploration, to find what exercise you will do."

Ugh. Nothing sounds good except going to bed with some candy.

"Maybe you would enjoy a class with friends, like Zumba," he suggests.

I am not going to any class with all those skinnies when I am still this size.

"Or maybe you could try yoga. The DVDs available for beginners and for advanced students are as abundant as the classes," he says.

I will think about that. Maybe I could try a DVD in the privacy of my bedroom with my computer. At least, it is an idea I don't terribly hate.

"There is not a right exercise for everyone, Young Jackie. Pilates, weight training, tennis, boot camp. The trick is finding what you will consistently do. Do not be married necessarily to one exercise," he says. "For a season, you may like swimming. Then, weight lifting. Then boot camp classes, and then yoga by yourself with DVDs. It does not matter what you do as long as you exercise consistently. Some women are routine lovers and do one thing forever. Other women enjoy change and variety, so they mix it up."

"I guess I could try walking and also working out to DVDs in my bedroom for now," I suggest. And when I get a little thinner, I think I would like to try weight lifting in a gym. Weight training has always interested me, but I would not know where to start with all those complicated machines.

"Remember, Young Jackie, you can have *excuses or results*, but not both," he says.

The mind-set that I can have *results without much work* continues to get shattered.

"You now know you should exercise because of the benefits," he says. "And you now know to make an appointment with yourself on your calendar. You have selected an exercise to try. Now, we have to *get ready*. If you are walking, then you need the appropriate clothes, good shoes, a visor, and sunscreen. Do you have a friend lined up to walk with? Or instead, what about having good music on your phone with earphones, ready to use? If you are going to try yoga on a DVD, you will need to buy it as well as purchase a mat. Whatever you are going to try, you need to plan and get ready. No plan, no exercise."

This guy keeps saying that if I fail to plan, then I should plan to fail. Sigh.

"If you plan to exercise in the morning," he says, "then to add Willpower Points to the morning, get your clothes out the night before, pack your lunch the night before, get your clothes out for work the night before, so you will have more morning minutes. If you do this, the likelihood of following through on your exercise grows."

"Gosh, Genie, you just added an hour to my evening routine," I say.

"Yes, when we make new goals and set priorities, schedules have to change," he says.

"Genie, does any woman do all this?" I ask.

"Of course they do," he says. "But after exercise becomes a habit, you will not have to expend so much energy. That is the great thing about habits: they tend to carry you like a mighty current."

My mighty current at the moment is watching a movie on Netflix.

"Your friends will try to convince you to do what works for then," he says. "You must find out what works for *you*. Maybe you would like going to the gym. Maybe you would like to bike. Or watch TV while walking on a treadmill. Finding the right exercise is extremely important as no one will consistently do something they hate."

But I hate it all.

"Your Demanding Child will fight you, so be ready for her sabotaging thoughts, such as 'Aw, this is hard and uncomfortable.' Instead, prior to exercise, read the list of benefits that I quoted for you earlier. Tell your Demanding Child that maybe it is hard for a few minutes, but the benefits are worth it. Read and reread your lists of the benefits of exercise, highlighting the ones that motivate you the most."

None of those benefits motivate me right now. I want chocolate and to go to sleep.

"Start small," he suggests. "Try ten minutes a day, three times a week. Then go up one minute per workout until you are exercising at least thirty minutes a day, most days. The accrued lifetime benefits of regularly exercising are inestimable."

Maybe I could start with ten minutes a day, three times a week. That is not too overwhelming.

"And do not forget the power of music," he says. "Music will transport you to another place. Turn on the upbeat music that you love. Everyone has music they love. Find and enjoy yours."

Beth has Pandora on her phone that she uses for working out. Maybe I could download that app onto my smart phone.

Again, this comes down to me. Am I willing to do the hard work of *change*? Everybody hates change. The brain hates change. At least he says I can start with ten minutes, three times a week. I can do that. At least, I think I can. I don't have any excuses not to.

"Today we talked about the basics of getting started exercising," the Genie says. "Later, after exercise becomes a habit for you, you can go online and learn about interval training and weight lifting, which not only will change your hormones from fat storing to fat burning, but will also rebuild muscle mass, which heightens your metabolic rate. But that is too much new information for today."

Barely seeing myself walk ten minutes a day, three times a week, I certainly do not want any intense exercise program to begin.

"Exercise will eventually become a ritual, like brushing your teeth. What you will find, Young Jackie, is that you will not really feel great unless you have exercised that day. You control your weight by *what* you put in your mouth, by *how much* you put in your mouth, and by *how much* you move."

Why cannot reading burn a lot of calories?

"I want to warn you that your Demanding Child does not want to push herself or be uncomfortable," he says. "Know that on most days, you will encounter the resistance of your Demanding Child when it is time to exercise. One of my former *Skinny School* students used to talk out loud to her Demanding Child when her Demanding Child showed up with her daily resistance to exercise. She would say 'Good morning, Demanding Child. Of course, you showed up with resistance. That is what you do; you try to get me to do what is *easiest* now, not what is *best* now. Today, I will plan *what and when* as far as my exercise. Exercise is a nonnegotiable for me since I want to be thin and healthy. The benefits of exercise are unparalleled. I will bathe my mind with the benefits of exercise and will get started, even if you, my Demanding Child, are screaming not to.'"

Oh, dear. Another cockamamie idea. He wants me to talk to myself?

"Demanding Child is always in the shadows, ready to convince you to take the immediate path of ease and comfort now," he says. "You must be ready for her incessant backstabbing."

I know her tactics. They have worked well for years.

"Bottom line, you will probably have to deal with the resistance of Demanding Child *every day the rest of your life* as far as exercise. So to counteract that, you have to bathe the Sane Adult portion of your brain with the benefits and reasons why you must schedule and plan exercise, or else it will not get done. *It will never be easy, and you will rarely want to.* Overcoming the easy path that Demanding Child clamors for is a battle of your mind. Knowing you will fight your Demanding Child every day about exercise, you can plan strategy how to overcome her. Just like everyone enjoys dessert, but *Skinny School* students do not eat it because they want something else more, most women do not enjoy exercise—a few do—but they feel great *after it is over.* However, the benefits are so phenomenal that they plan, prep, and trick themselves into doing it using music, laying clothes out, meeting a friend, etcetera. The battle to exercise is before the exercise ever happens. It is in your mind that you *know* you must do it. The point is, you can often outsmart your psychological resistance with some clever thinking, such as getting out your gym clothes, visor, shoes, etcetera, the night before."

Ugh. Exercise. Ugh.

"We have now concluded Part I of *Skinny School,* Young Jackie. You have learned all nine secrets that are nonnegotiable for being permanently thin. When I return, we will begin Advanced Training, in which I will teach you strategies for special situations. There are new workout clothes hanging in your closet, as well as ingredients prepped in your fridge for a Genie Vegetable Omelet in the morning," he says, and he disintegrates.

Hearing my text message beep, I assume it is from Brandon, saying something sappy, such as he hopes we can be friends or some other such nonsense.

Oh, my gosh, it is from Zach.

Why did you leave early? Are you home? Are you free? I need a friend to talk to.

I write back: **We left early because I had to talk to Brandon about something. And yes, I am home and free.**

Can I come over and we go for a drive so we can talk?

This is strange. Reeeeally strange.

Sure, I write.

Is 15 minutes okay? he texts.

Zach arrives in almost exactly fifteen minutes. Getting in his car, I'm nervous, wondering what he wants to talk about. Zach is never one to give away his emotions, but I can tell he is agitated.

"Rachel and I had a fight on the way home, and I need someone to help me think," he begins, even before we are out of the parking lot of my apartment complex. Zach's mild manners and calm spirit are not usually ruffled, but tonight, they are.

I want to say, "That is what snakes do, Zach—they bite," but I use my self-control instead.

"As soon as we left the wedding," he begins, "she accused me of not being attentive to her. She said I did not notice when she needed another refill of her drink and that I walked around and talked to everyone but her. And last, she said she thought I should take dance lessons."

Zach is a pretty terrible dancer, but really, even a prince in shining armor cannot be perfect. I look at this mountain of a man, obviously shaken. At the moment, he seems more like a little puppy who just got sprayed by a fire hose.

Zach glances over at me to see if I am listening. Noting that I am, he continues.

"Should it be this hard, Jack? I mean, I know relationships are messy, but should it be *this* hard?"

Wanting to say every single mean thing I can about Rachel, I am pricked by an invisible feeling that warns me not to. Instead, I feel obligated to talk to Zach as I would a best friend.

"All relationships have to go *through conflict to get to intimacy*," I tell Zach, something my sister Jessica has taught me. "Maybe this is a conflict you need to work through."

I cannot believe I am saying this. I want to say, *Bag that wretch*. Instead, I am encouraging him to stay in the relationship and see if they can work it out.

Zach drives to a neighborhood park, and we sit on a picnic table and talk for another twenty minutes. Zach has visibly calmed down. "I guess you are right," he says. "Conflict is a part of every relationship, so I need to see if we can work through this. Jack, I appreciate it. I knew you would help me think through this." We walk back to his car to drive to my apartment complex. The counseling session is over.

Zach leaves, and I stand on my porch, knowing I said the right thing. Not listening to my lower nature tonight, I gave Zach the right advice, even though it was painful and difficult to do.

The stars are beautiful as I gaze up toward the night sky. Realizing that the advice I gave Zach was not my own, but Someone Else's, there is a strange peace in my heart. My heart feels broken, shredded, and alone. However, I know I am *not* alone. My faith is my Rock.

Walking into my closet before I crawl into bed, I notice my new, hip workout clothes. I gather my shoes, visor, and sunglasses for an early-morning walk. I like the idea of walking and praying, and man, do I need to do some praying.

The nonnegotiables in *Skinny School* so far are:

1. I expect to work like a Champion to retrain my mind since this is a Top Four Life Goal.
2. Ditching sweets and starches is not optional if I want to overhaul my metabolism. I am to track my sugar/carb grams as well as my calories.

I focus on all the beautiful, delicious food *I get to eat* instead of what I must not eat.

3. Planning and prepping are the secrets Champions use to conquer goals. I must daily make Quart Bags.

4. Hunger is my friend, and waiting until I am truly hungry and quitting before I am full are nonnegotiable. Tracking my hunger is imperative and will expose how I deceive myself with wanting to eat for self-soothing and entertainment.

5. By listing the schemes of Demanding Child in my Ruby Journal and accessing how my Sane Adult really feels, I can dismantle the Demanding Child's tricks, one by one.

6. Failure can be useful, if I will evaluate it and learn from it.

7. Finding substitutes for soothing and entertaining myself besides using food is imperative. Discovering my passion and immersing myself in it will be extremely healing to my food obsession.

8. A clean environment, one without Trash Food, is crucial to reduce temptation.

9. Daily I will face resistance to exercise. Therefore, I must plan and prep my exercise like Champions do to accomplish their current Top Four Life Goals.

Advanced Training

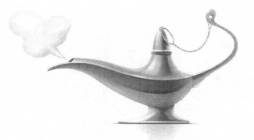

Lesson 10

Understand the Influence of
Your Social Circles

Thursday, October 2   Weight: 159   Pounds lost: 16   Still to lose: 29

I tell Tory she has to move out and she says fine, that Brandon has a garage apartment that she can move into until she gets financially on her own. What she should have said is, "until I get financially *on* Brandon." I feel sorry for him, but hey, I cannot solve the problems of the universe. He wants her beauty; she wants his money. I will never see that $750 she owes me, but cutting the cords with Tory feels so great, so freeing. Finally, I will come home to a clean kitchen and my brown suede boots will be in my closet.

And I am through with Gramps, thank goodness, but that means, no surprise, I am alone again. That is my go-to status: *alone.*

Zach is now trying to work through his conflict with Rachel and her issues. Seeing that all couples have issues, he will probably propose soon. Obviously, I am jealous out of my mind of Rachel's skinniness and her well-bred parentage. She is probably not a snob to anyone else—just nobody me.

"Good morning, Zach," I cheerfully say as I arrive at the office. He is already at his desk.

"Good morning," he says in a low voice. That is not the usual tone for Zach, so I pause in the doorway.

"Everything okay?" I ask.

He looks up but not with his normal expression. "The other side in the Montgomery case got a summary judgment. I just read the e-mail."

In law, when the other side gets a summary judgment, that means the judge thinks the case you are bringing is no good, and it is thrown out. I am very familiar with the Montgomery case and know what a low blow this is to Zach. Watching, I see him gloomily look at his computer screen. How rare for Zach to be down like this.

"Zach, losing a case does not mean you are a *crummy* lawyer. Losing a case means you are not a *perfect* lawyer. You are still a *great* lawyer."

He glances up and shakes his head in the smallest of ways. I guess I am being annoying and he wants to get back to work. Walking to my desk, I begin the new week's work.

Two hours later, Zach walks out of his office and hands me some documents to scan into the computer. We discuss a deposition and a Benefit Review Conference coming up. Starting to return to his office, he instead turns and says, "It amazes me how you know what other people are thinking, Jack. Earlier, you said that losing a case does not mean I am a crummy lawyer. Well, that was exactly what I was thinking, *that I was a crummy lawyer.* And then for you to reframe the thoughts, that losing a case only means I am not a *perfect* lawyer, but that I am still a *good* lawyer…well…that was very helpful."

"I said you are still a *great* lawyer," I correct him. That slight boyish grin flashes across his face.

"Thanks, Jack," and he returns to his desk.

My sister Jessica has made a similar remark to me before as the one Zach just made. Once she asked me, "How do you always know what other people are thinking?" I guess even we fatties have some good qualities.

Mrs. Simpson walks in after lunch because she wants Eva to make copies for her Garden Club committee notes as well as she wanted to drop off some gourmet fudge from the Nashville Candy Store for the office staff. Great. Just what I need.

Saying hello to her, I walk on by, but not without first getting a whiff of her breath. Obviously she has been drinking alcohol. Handsome, successful

Attorney Simpson has some ugly bones in those closets in his house, I am afraid.

The copy machine is in a room not directly adjacent to my office but close enough that I can hear everything Mrs. Simpson is saying, considering that her lunch cocktails may have turned off the volume control of her voice. "Eva, the modeling school down the street is starting a new semester, and I think you should sign up. Why, my modeling days were the highlight of my life!" Mrs. Simpson, who is now sixty-five and fifty pounds overweight, is talking about her golden days when she used to model. There is something pitiful about it.

"Mom, I have told you, I am too short," Eva remarks.

"That is ridiculous," Mrs. Simpson says. "You are perfect for that job. Definitely, I think you should go for it." Maybe I am imagining this, but her words seem a tiny bit slurred. "And I will tell you something else you should go for, and that is Zach Boltz. Why, if I was in my twenties, I would not let that man out of my sight."

"Mom! Shh!" I hear Eva plead. Even I am embarrassed for Eva.

A loud *thud* sounds, and I hear papers spilling. "Oh, sorry, how clumsy of me. Let me pick up the papers," I hear a frazzled Mrs. Simpson say.

"I will get them," Eva says in an exasperated voice, and again I hear the shuffling of papers.

Mrs. Simpson does not even take a breath. "I read an article yesterday in a magazine that says you have to let men know you are interested, but slyly. Men do not like overt moves by women but subtle moves," she says.

"Stop it, Mom," Eva says. "Not here."

"You have got to learn the balancing act of encouraging him, yet making yourself a challenge," Mrs. Simpson says, again in her loud voice.

"Your copies are finished," Eva says. "Please excuse me a second while I answer that phone." I did not hear a phone ring, but Mrs. Simpson's cocktails may keep her from realizing that.

Mrs. Simpson then appears in my doorway. "Oh, hi, Jackie. I forgot which way I came in." Actually, this is pretty sad.

"The front door is out that door to the right," I say. Standing up, I point in the correct direction.

"My, my, child. *You have lost a lot of weight!* My goodness. How much have you lost?"

Grateful that the office is empty and that Zach is not hearing this, I squeak out, "Sixteen pounds."

"Well, you lose much more and you will be in the running for the handsome Zach Boltz, too," she says as she turns and walks down the hall. Before I can respond, Zach walks in behind her. If he heard her, he acts like he did not.

"I brought you some coffee, Zach," Eva says, entering the room with coffee for Zach, "with two creams and no sugar." Obviously overhearing her mother, Eva turns to me, "I knew you had lost a lot of weight, but I did not realize it was sixteen pounds. How much more do you want to lose?"

Zach is now hearing all of this. I hate this. I hate this so much. And Eva's attempt to have an intimate conversation about my weight is not going to happen. No freakin' way.

"I'm not sure, Eva. When are you leaving for the post office? I have some demand packages that need to go out today," I say, keeping my anger composed but sending a message that we will *not* be discussing my weight.

"Four o'clock," she says and leaves. The tension over the last twenty minutes is screaming in every part of my body, first with Mrs. Simpson's comment about me being in the running for Zach, and second, with Eva's invasive questions. I wonder how I am going to calm down and get back to work.

"Jack, when do you want to meet to discuss the Snelly brief?" Zach calls from his office. I am not ready to do anything but scream. Or maybe indulge in some sort of immediate mood changer. A Snickers bar would do nicely.

"Can we do it in thirty minutes?" I answer back. That would give me time to go make some vanilla caramel herbal tea to soothe myself, instead of the usual sugar/carb treat I have used to use to calm myself. Learning to turn down my emotional volume without Trash Food is a new lesson for me, one in which I have a long way to go. I hate emotional turbulence.

After getting up to brew some herbal tea, I then decide to take a walk around the block to soothe myself. I grab some veggies out of my Quart Bag to crunch down on, too. The gourmet fudge on the counter is calling my name, but somehow I manage to head out the door without grabbing a piece.

It is such a beautiful day, and I can feel that the walk and the veggies from my Quart Bags begin to comfort me. **Surprisingly, the Genie appears.** "No one can see or hear me but you, Young Jackie. Today I want to address *the influence that your social circles have on your eating*."

He picks the worst times to show up.

"Humans are very vulnerable to mimicking the behaviors of those around them," he begins. "I can tell you much about a person if I know whom they have coffee with."

What does having coffee with someone tell you?

"Humans were created to be community beings, and they are tremendously influenced by the people around them," he says. "Advertising and the surrounding culture influences humans, but nothing influences humans like the other humans they are in daily contact with."

So?

"Most humans think they are above the influence of others," he says, "but they are wrong. If the people that are in your inner circle value honesty, then you will have this tug to be honest. If the people in your inner group value serving others, then you likewise will be pulled in that direction. If those around you value materialism, you will have a tendency to mirror this value also. It is a cosmic law that humans influence other humans greatly."

Surely not me. I think I stand above this concept.

"If the people in your social circles eat healthy and value exercise," he says, "then you will be influenced to do the same. If the people in your social circles eat Trash Food, then your tendency will be to do likewise. I am not admonishing you to change people groups. I am only alerting you to raise your antennas when you are around others. If they constantly talk and think about Trash Food, then you will be drawn to do so also. If your friends and family discuss healthy eating, then this will be a positive influence on you."

Tory made chocolate-chip cookies; Mrs. Simpson brings fudge to the office; at church, they serve cookies and donuts; and Beth eats Hershey's Bars every day. I cannot think of one person in my social circle who truly cares about eating healthy.

"Just knowing that another person's habits and beliefs influence you will help you see the patterns if you begin to look for them," he says. "If you are going to a wedding shower at which you know that the hostesses will only serve food choices that are full of sugar and refined carbs, then you can prepare and bring yourself a little bag of nuts. *Being mentally prepared* is your mantra, Young Jackie. You must prepare yourself against the influence of even your closest friends if they have a lifestyle of ingesting sugar and refined carbs."

"So what do I say to them?" I ask.

"You do not need to say anything," he says. "I am not suggesting you lecture them or call them out about their poor food habits. I am only suggesting that you gird up *your own mind* so that you can see what is happening and not fall into eating Trash Food, just because the people around you eat it. Hopefully someday your friends will notice your change in lifestyle and will eventually ask you for your advice. Then you can be a positive influence on them."

Ha-ha, that's funny. Me, the chub, influencing others to eat right.

"I have left you a batch of Genie Deviled Eggs in your refrigerator at your apartment," he says and disappears.

As I walk back to my desk, Zach hears me and asks if I am ready to begin working on the Snelly case. Feeling pleasantly restored emotionally, I say okay, but first I freshen my lipstick and powder. I like my coral shirt over these slimming gray slacks with this beautiful scarf. Maybe Zach will notice.

Not looking up from his paperwork when I enter his office, Zach begins talking. "I have a deposition scheduled in the Johnston case in Boca Raton in four weeks, and I could use help organizing the documents and paperwork during the deposition. Attorney Simpson authorized you to go with me. We would fly down on Sunday evening, November ninth, for the deposition on the tenth and eleventh. Do you have a conflict?"

Go on a business trip with Zach? Just me? The thought so delights me that I tell myself to act calm and cool. It is easy to forget that Zach has a girlfriend and that he will soon propose.

"Go to Boca Raton where it is seventy-five degrees in November? I might be able to talk myself into that," I say, acting like it is the weather that excites me, instead of sitting by him on the plane, riding with him in the cab, and eating a few meals alone with him.

"This is my biggest case, and this deposition means everything to the case," he says. I know this is business to him, but it is ecstasy to me.

Walking back to my desk, I find that my thoughts are anywhere but on my work. What I am thinking about is how much more weight I can lose before that trip…and that then I need to buy a bunch of new clothes!

Note to Reader: The Nine Nonnegotiables for Skinny School are in Appendix B at the back of this book.

Lesson 11

Slaying the Hog-Wild Mentality

Friday, October 17   *Weight: 155*   *Pounds lost: 20*   *Still to lose: 25*

Zach and I attended a Benefit Review Conference this morning, and by his demeanor, I can tell he does not think it went well. Not to mention that the conference took two hours longer than it should have because the other lawyer was trying to stretch out the time, since he gets paid hourly. We are now headed back to the office. I wish Zach would mention stopping for lunch, but he does not.

His text sound beeps, and he checks his phone at the stoplight. He breathes a big sigh.

"What is wrong?" I ask.

"It is my mother," he says. "She is out of town, and my grandmother, who lives at a retirement home, needs her blood pressure medicine picked up. The retirement home usually takes residents to do these errands, but Grandma missed her ride. Grandma says she is completely out of her medicine and needs it today." He sighs again. Knowing Zach, he is not irritated that he needs to help his grandmother. He is merely frustrated over his perceived failure at the Benefit Review Conference along with the extra two hours he spent at the event. Now this task is going to put him farther behind.

"Where are the retirement home and the pharmacy?" I ask.

"Not far from here," Zach says.

"Well, let's go," I say.

He glances over and catches my eye. I can tell he does not want to spend the thirty or forty-five minutes doing this, but if I know Zach, we are now on our way to the pharmacy.

"I know you also have a lot of work to do at the office, so I am sorry about this," he says.

"I like old people," I say and smile. And it is true. Old people rock.

Zach nods. He is not in a very playful mood.

We turn around, and soon we are at the Walgreens drive-through, picking up his grandmother's prescription. An older lady behind the glass window speaks over the microphone, "Your grandmother just called. She said that a very handsome lawyer would soon be picking up her blood pressure medicine."

"All grandmothers feel the duty to inflate the image of their grandchildren, and mine is no different," Zach replies. The cashier smiles, but I know she is thinking it is no inflation.

We arrive at the Blakeford retirement home, and Zach asks if I would like to wait in the car. "Are you kidding me? Retirement homes are the best," I say as I hop out of the car.

"My grandmother is hard of hearing, so you have to speak up so she can hear you," he warns me.

I nod.

There are many eighty- and ninety-year-olds everywhere, chatting loudly so their friends can hear them. Many of the residents have walkers. I see a humpbacked lady with gorgeous, thick gray hair piled high on her head walk toward us. "Zachy! Zachy!" she says, as she hobbles toward us.

"Zachy?" I say, a little under my breath, but loud enough so he can hear. He raises his eyebrows and whispers back, "It is better than Boo Boo, which is what she calls my brother." And he walks toward her to hug her.

"I forgot my hearing aid, Zachy, so you will have to speak extra loudly," she says. Her face is smooth, and her eyes twinkle. Immediately I like her.

Zach loudly says, "Grandma, this is Jackie, my new legal assistant."

"Oh, you are Zachy's new love interest?" she asks. "Why, that is so nice." She steps back and examines me, as if she examining a dress she might purchase. She immediately lowers her voice, "I never liked that snooty little girl that Zach has been toting around. You look so much more pleasant, child. Are you from Nashville, dear?"

I look at Zach for help, but he simply shrugs his shoulders.

Loudly I say, "I am Zach's *legal assistant*."

"Louisiana? I have an aunt in Louisiana. That is a good state. Yes, yes, she is fine, Zachy. I really like her. I like her eyes. I always say you can tell a lot about a person through their eyes, and this girl is fine. That bag of bones that you used to bring here had dark eyes. I did not want to tell you while you were still dating her, Zachy, but I knew I could not trust her. Now this girl, she has a little meat on her. I like a little meat on the bones. Curves, that is what we used to call it."

Fat is what I call it.

Zach is exceptionally quiet. I think he realizes he is helpless in this situation.

"Grandma, do you need anything else? I need to get back to my office," Zach says in a loud voice.

"Have you set a date?" she asks.

Zach has had enough.

"Grandma, this is my legal assistant. She *works* for me," he tries again.

"Oh, you're *waiting* awhile. Good choice. I always say you should wait awhile because it takes a little time for the warts to rise to the surface. But just do not wait too long, Zachy. Your grandma wants to be able to walk down the aisle in your wedding, and I am ninety next month."

Giving up, Zach hugs and kisses his grandmother good-bye. She reaches for me to hug me, too. "Welcome to the family, honey. You are just a delight. An absolute delight. I am a good judge of people, and Zachy did a good job choosing this time!"

I hug her back and smile, and we leave.

Both of us are quiet as we get into the car.

"I guess a hearing aid is a pretty important device when you get that age," I say, trying to make light of the situation.

But Zach does not respond. I am pretty sure he is bothered by what Grandma said about Rachel and her dark eyes.

I certainly like Grandma. She and I have very similar opinions.

Zach takes a call from a client and we soon arrive back at the office where, as usual, Zach and I grind out the work until it is time to leave.

Driving home to my apartment, I feel lonely as I realize it is Friday night and I have nothing planned to do. **Walking in, however, I find the Genie in my kitchen, and he is in great spirits.** He has prepared a delicious dish of mahi-mahi, a romaine salad with tiny-chopped vegetables, and green beans with Dijon lemon butter waiting on me.

"Young Jackie, tonight's topic is called Slaying the Hog-Wild Mentality. This mentality is a trick that your Demanding Child uses that must be confronted. You are human, and you certainly are going to err once in a while on your program. Maybe you eat a piece of bread. Maybe you eat fries off a friend's plate. These little errors are not ideal, but *they lead to a Hog-Wild Mentality.*"

Lead to what?

"Your Demanding Child whispers to you, 'You have messed up, so you might as well enjoy yourself.' You see, Demanding Child is always looking for tricks so she can enjoy herself *right now.* After listening to her, you say to yourself, 'Yes, I have messed up, so I may as well go Hog Wild and eat whatever I want.' That is exactly what Demanding Child wants. However, what was maybe a few chips at a Mexican restaurant has now turned into a three-thousand-calorie binge. Do you see the insanity of this?"

Uh...I see that I think like this.

"This is a big point, Young Jackie. After you eat a few bites of something not on your program, *get hold of yourself.* It is only a little mishap. Your Demanding Child is waiting in the wings, so she can convince you to pull out the stops and really 'enjoy' this moment. That is her constant drum beat: *enjoy yourself right this second.* How harmful to your true goals she is! Your only defense is to have your mind prepped to such an extent that you realize how she is *constantly trying to sabotage you.* Your mind must be on hyper-alert, so you will recognize her insidious strategies and therefore be able to resist her with your Sane Adult's thinking."

That is exactly what happens to me. I mess up a little and then go Hog Wild, thinking I will start over tomorrow.

"If you do mess up a little, realize it and immediately, right now, this moment, not later, this second...get back on the bus! Ditch sweets and starches, track your food, be sure you have planned and prepped food available, read your Ruby Journal, and for sure, wait until you are physically hungry to eat!"

The basics of *Skinny School*, of course. *Ditch, plan, and wait.*

"And as I said in Lesson Six on failure, do not waste this incidence. Do not fret over it, but record it. Learn from it. And then, get back on the bus—your *Skinny School* program—before you do some real damage."

How does he know all my little habits? Do other women act as insane as I do? I do feel better knowing that my behavior is not crazy and that it is, in his opinion, fixable.

"If a woman goes off her plan," he says, "the very moment she realizes what she is doing, she must stop, record what tripped her up—what ploy her Demanding Child used to throw her off her program—and then say to herself, 'Enough of that.' No Hog-Wild Eating. What an insane, ridiculous idea that you will start tomorrow instead of immediately drawing a line in the sand and saying, 'That craziness is over.' Do not let Demanding Child trick you."

Hog-Wild Eating and I are old chums, for sure.

"Watch out for when your Demanding Child says, 'What the heck! I already botched it. So I may as well go to town and live it up.' Your Demanding Child will have many different sentences to get you off your program."

What I thought was a serious neurosis in my mind is simply something that all humans have, a Demanding Child personality! All I have to do is to alert myself to her schemes. Wow, I might be able to do that.

"The next time you slip up and hear your Demanding Child tell you to go Hog Wild, you will have a strategy ready. The strategy is you say no, get some herbal tea—and your Quart Bags, if you must—and move into the *Miraculous Threesome*: Ditch, Plan, Wait. However, even now, your failure from earlier is not wasted, since we recorded and evaluated it in your Ruby Journal."

His other students must have been Superwoman and Wonder Woman, not mere mortals.

"I have left some Genie Deli Turkey Bacon Rollups in your fridge for the next time you are a three," he says, and he evaporates. My cell rings, and it is Beth.

"Guess what?" she says. "Rachel's dad owns a booth at the Titans stadium. Richard, Zach, Rachel, and I are all going this Sunday afternoon to the game. Rachel's cousin, Will, from Kansas, is visiting, and Rachel suggested you go with us to make it a six-some."

Rachel is fixing me up with her cousin? Maybe she is softening to me after all. I immediately remember what Zach's grandmother said today about Rachel's dark eyes. The temptation to tell Beth is huge, but I resist.

"What do you know about her cousin?" I ask.

"I do not know much," Beth says. "All Rachel said was that he works in the family business. We are going together in Rachel's mother's Suburban, so we can all ride together. We will pick you up at noon on Sunday if that is okay." No matter how bad this might be, Beth will be there, so I agree to go.

We hang up, and I feel better. Knowing I have plans on Sunday afternoon with a blind date—no less Rachel's cousin—helps my self-pity at being alone on a Friday night. Well, I might just head to the mall to get something new and cute to wear! Things may be turning around for me after all.

Lesson 12

Dialing Down Emotional Tidal Waves

Sunday, October 19   Weight: 154   Pounds lost: 21   Still to lose: 24

Having trouble finding something I want to wear to church this morning, I am rather late and have difficulty finding a seat. I sit by a single guy who introduces himself as Brad. He is a little squirrely looking but nice enough.

Hustling home after the service, I change clothes and get ready for my blind date with high-class Rachel's cousin. What a compliment that she thinks I would be good enough for her cousin! Maybe the past is really going to be the past.

Beth texts me: **Get your expectations down very low, Jackie. I am not impressed at all with Will. Sorry.**

What is wrong with him? I text back. I mean, how bad could he be?

I am not sure but he is a little off. You will see.

Hearing a knock at the door, I open it. The guy standing there has a funny look on his face. "Jackie?" he asks. He starts laughing and snorting. I can immediately tell there is something not quite right. I am not sure what, but he has a screw loose or something.

Will and I get into the Suburban, and Rachel is very friendly. "Hey, Jackie! Nice to see you," but Zach is extraordinarily quiet.

Beth and Richard try to keep the conversation light and funny, but we all now know that Rachel set me up with her cousin who is a little *off.* He has some mental disability. I am not a snob, and I will certainly act nice, but for Rachel to fix me up with someone with clear mental issues is...well, hurtful.

Arriving at the suite at the Titans Stadium, I try to talk to Will about the Titans, but his inappropriate laugh and his lack of understanding are obvious. He is definitely a little disturbed in some capacity.

"So you work in your family business?" I politely ask.

"I guess," he says and again cackles loudly and inappropriately. "I run errands and vacuum." He snickers again, as if that was truly a very funny sentence.

Breathing deeply, I walk back to the food area to get a refill on my drink. Zach and Rachel are behind a partition and do not know I can hear them. "I cannot believe you fixed Will up with Jackie," Zach says. "You did not tell me he had a mental disability."

"Oh," she retorted, "so now you are judging him for having a low IQ?"

"Of course not, Rachel," Zach says. "You know me better than that. But Jackie is brilliant, and she is not going to be romantically interested in someone that is mentally impaired. It is such an obvious mismatch."

"I know you like Jackie, Zach, but she is fat, and fat girls cannot be choosy in whom they date," she says.

I quickly and quietly return to my seat, so no one will know I overheard. My stomach feels like I was the one on the field who just got tackled and slammed. I am so ill feeling that I want to throw up. Rachel is as mean as ever. She thinks my weight means I am desperate enough that I would date someone with a mental impairment. I am not a snob, and of course I have compassion for people with mental handicaps. But that does not mean I am involved romantically with them. The nerve of her. How can a prince like Zach put up with her beastliness?

The game is over, and Rachel suggests we all go back to her apartment to play cards. I say I have a stomachache—which is not a lie—and probably should go home. Zach again gives me a look of compassion. Will says we should stop and get some Pepto-Bismol. He tells the group how it helps him when he has diarrhea. The fun is out of the group, as everybody feels the tension.

The group drops me off, and I want to medicate my anger at Rachel. Her words ring in my ears: *She is fat, and fat girls cannot be choosy in whom they date.* My text message sound beeps. It is from Zach.

I am very sorry about the blind date. I had no prior information about Will. I apologize for Rachel's error. I know you were uncomfortable.

Zach is trying to be sweet, but the pain is deep and sharp. He does not even know I heard the remark, *fat girls cannot be choosy in whom they date.*

I write, I know you were not involved in that matchmaking. Thanks for your concern, Zach.

Rachel's words play over and over again in my ears. *Fat girls cannot be choosy in whom they date.* Rachel thinks that since I have a weight problem, I am in some subcategory of human being. The superiority she feels to me is cutting and agonizing. Rachel is the type of person that I must remember to stay as far away from as I can. She is just plain hateful.

A cloud of depression descends upon me. Nothing feels good. Nothing feels hopeful. I only want this pain to go away, and the only way I know to quickly accomplish that is with food. Thoughts of what Trash Food I could eat start to download into my brain.

"Hello, Young Jackie," says the high-energy voice of the Genie. "Today is the perfect day to discuss the topic of Dialing Down Emotional Tidal Waves."

Nothing like matching the topic to the situation.

"In the past when you have had severe emotional distress, you learned to dial down the discomfort with Trash Food. Actually, that strategy works: the discomfort immediately decreases. But eating large amounts of Trash Food to medicate unpleasant feelings does not get you what you really want, as you well know."

Sometimes, I don't care. I want the pain to go away.

"There are several strategies that have worked well for my *Skinny School* clients in the past. Ultimately, the answer to this issue is to learn to think differently about unwanted circumstances, and thus the huge emotional reaction will be less. But for now, since you are having escalated emotional feelings to unwanted situations, we need a strategy."

He is dang right I need a strategy, or I am driving through a fast-food restaurant and ordering two of everything.

"The first thing you should reach for are your Quart Bags," the Genie says. "The chomping can be lifesaving in these instances. If the Quart Bags are not enough to dial down your feelings, try eating something like two apples and three eggs. This is *eating when you are* not *hungry,* and it is *not* ideal, but we are dealing with a tsunami emotional tidal wave, and we have to adjust the rules. We are trying to prevent a three-thousand-calorie binge. So fill up on the food I just mentioned. Then get your mind on something else. If you have a novel you like, immerse yourself in reading. If you have a game you like to play on your iPad or phone, that will give your mind something else to focus on also. But you must find something else for your mind to think about because that is what will dial down the mental turmoil. Call a friend, take a walk or a bath, read a magazine—or do all of these strategies. Just know that the desire to tone down upsetting emotions with Trash Food has been your strategy in the past, and now you know that you can replace that habit with these new suggestions."

"I don't know if I can. The discomfort is so intense," I say.

"Maybe you cannot the first time, but you will be able to the second time, or the third time, or even the fourth. *Skinny School* is a program where you learn, and you are not expected to be perfect. What usually happens with any diet program is *that the participant fails and then chucks the whole program.* Heavens, please do not do that. You will mess up on the *Skinny School* program, but do not throw the program out. *Champions persevere in their goals, even though they initially might meet with failure.* Write about the failure in your Ruby Journal, learn from it, and get back on the bus! When you realize that failure is part of this program—as it is with any new learning endeavor— then you can forgive yourself, learn the lesson you need, and get right back on your program. Not tomorrow. Now. This second. Eventually, *if you will continue to come back to this program,* you will all of a sudden, *flip your switch.* You will say to yourself, 'I am terribly upset, but I am going to get my Quart Bags, two apples, some protein, and a novel, then run a bath and try to dial down how I am feeling.'"

My emotions are already somewhat dissipating. Not completely but somewhat. I do see how his strategy might work. I am not used to dialing down my emotions with anything except Trash Food, but I do have a glimmer of hope that I could learn another strategy.

The Genie departs but leaves a recipe for a Genie Veggie Omelet on the counter, along with the necessary ingredients: bell peppers, spinach, mushrooms, onions, eggs, and cheese.

Many text messages came in while the Genie was here. One from my sister Jessica, wanting to know about the date. One message was from Beth, talking about how ridiculous that was of Rachel to fix me up with Will. Another from my other sister Chloe, who heard from Jessica about the blind date. And last, another text from Zach, asking if I am okay and if my stomach is really hurting.

Simultaneously I write each of them back while I sauté vegetables to put into an omelet. I text Beth, I text Zach, I text Chole, and now I am going to text Jessica last.

My omelet is almost done. I watch it closely to make sure it does not burn while I finish texting everyone back.

I text to Jessica: **Not only did Rachel intentionally fix me up with her cousin, knowing he has a mental impairment, but I also heard her tell Zach that "fat girls cannot be choosy in whom they date." I cannot believe Zach dates that villainous thing.**

Oh, my! My omelet is getting overdone. I click SEND and quickly get the omelet out of the skillet.

Sitting down to eat my eggs, something feels a little wrong. I glance at my phone and my heart stops. What did I just do? Oh, my, goodness. I meant to send that last message to Jessica, but I accidentally sent it to Zach. Oh. My. Double. Goodness. Surely, I didn't. I didn't. I couldn't have.

But I did. I reread what I sent Zach. No. No. Oh, heavens, no!

The text message beeps. Of course, it is from Zach. **Did you mean to send that to me?**

I breathe deeply and wish I could die. I wish I could lie down in the grave and pull the dirt up over my head. I will never get past this. I called Rachel "a villainous thing." Oh, could I please wake up from this nightmare?

I do not know what to do except own it. I text: **That text was for my sister Jessica. I accidentally sent it to you. Of course you know how embarrassed I am now. That was wrong of me to call Rachel a "villainous thing." I apologize.**

He quickly writes back: **I was very disappointed that Rachel said that about you. And now I am sad that you heard and were hurt. She was wrong to say that. I hope you will be able to forgive her.**

Forgive her? I don't want to forgive her. I want to slander her and pray down all sorts of curses on her. I want her to be miserable, like she made me today.

The anxiety is clanging. The despair of the day is horrible. After eating my semi-burned omelet, I grab a cup of hot vegetable soup and my Quart Bags of celery, romaine lettuce, and cherry tomatoes, make some hot tea, and run a big bath of hot water, getting out my Michael Connelly novel to take me away to another world. I hate life at this moment. I hate fatness; I hate snobby, skinny, country club girls. I hate almost everything. Getting into a tub of overflowing bubbles, I open my book to try to change my deep despair. The Genie was not exaggerating when he said I needed a strategy for Emotional Tidal Waves. This is a full-blown tsunami.

Lesson 13

Overcoming Nighttime Eating

Monday, October 27   *Weight: 152*   *Pounds lost: 23*   *Still to lose: 22*

Weeks ago I was supposed to start training Eva to become a legal assistant, but as normal, things got in the way. Therefore, today is the lucky (choke choke) day that Attorney Simpson decides that we will begin the training. With Zach's new cases, my work load is at an unusually high volume, but I take a deep breath and prepare for my unpleasant task ahead.

The Barbie doll walks into my office. Truly, she is a study in fashion. She has on a short camel skirt with a cream sweater. Her brown boots are flat and tightly hug her calves, leaving quite a few inches between them and the skirt. She has a huge brown, gold, camel, and cream scarf wrapped around her neck, and her hair is piled high on her head. Altogether, including the boots, she probably weighs 110 pounds. Disgusting.

Eva and I begin to discuss the computer program Amicus, in which our law firm stores all of its information about our cases. "How do you get into the Amicus program again? I cannot remember where to click," she says. After three explanations, I'm getting a little weary.

Attorney Simpson walks in with some papers for Zach. "Hi, Daddy," she chirps. "I am learning the Amicus program."

Yeah, at about the speed at which chimpanzees would learn, I might add.

Attorney Simpson glances over at me to get my feedback. "We are progressing, sir," I say.

Zach walks out of his office to take the papers from Attorney Simpson, and as stiff faced as Zach usually is, I think I perceive the teeniest of grins. After he takes the papers from Attorney Simpson, the men go out in the hall to talk.

That miniscule smile was worth a department store full of Michael Kors shoes and purses. It said, *I know you are hating this, and they do not get it but I do.* Yes, Zach said all of that in that one little quarter-fraction of a smile. What it means to a woman to feel understood! Zach is the last person to talk ill of others (I am working on my tongue, though), but he wanted to communicate to me, *I know that training Eva is taxing you.* Maybe I am taking this too far, but a little, tiny smile can change another person's perspective...if it is from the right person.

"Daddy," Eva calls to her dad in the hall, "I need to leave early today. I'm getting highlights in my hair."

"Sure, honey," says Attorney Simpson, and he returns to his office.

Eva's text message beeps, and all I can read is the top, which says the sender's name is Chad. This is a new guy that I have not heard about. "That is enough for today," Eva says as she gets up from the computer. Immediately she begins to click, click, click and return the text. Since I have a brief to work on, demand packages to get out, and umpteen letters to write, I'm relieved our training session is over.

Eva abruptly returns. "Oh, guys," she says loudly enough so Zach can hear too, "I'm having a Halloween party next Thursday night. Can you both come? Zach, can you bring Rachel?"

I hate Halloween parties. That means the skinny girls will be there as Catwoman, and the chunks like me will be there as the witches from *Harry Potter*, wearing long, drapey robes.

"I think we can," Zach says. "I will ask Rachel."

She looks at me to get a response. What do I say? I cannot say the truth, which is, *I am still too fat to enjoy costume parties.*

Smiling, I say, "Sure, sounds like fun." What actresses fat chicks have to become.

Zach walks to the door that separates our offices. "When do you want to get organized for the Somerville brief?" he asks.

"When is good for you?" I ask. We lock eyes, even though we are only talking business.

"I need to go visit a new client in the hospital," he says. "How do you feel about riding with me and discussing the brief on the way there?"

Gulp. These trips alone in the car with Zach throw me. At least I wore this new cute outfit. "I could do that," I say, trying not to act too excited.

"Since Eva already left," he continues, "how do you feel about first taking this certified letter to the post office? Then you can text me when you are back, and I will come out to the car." Zach is always the ultra efficient one, saving minutes everywhere.

"That will work," I say in a friendly voice. Zach returns to his office, and for some reason, the memory of last Sunday at the Titans game appears in my head. Rachel's words ring in my ear: *I know you like Jackie, Zach, but she is fat, and fat girls cannot be choosy whom they date.* Realizing how ridiculous it is to let negative thoughts and memories throw me into a wad, I try to think about something else.

Driving to the post office, I mail Zach's letter and head back to the office. **The Genie abruptly appears in my passenger seat.** I am not too happy to see him, however, as I wanted to freshen my makeup in the car before I am alone with Zach, and I only have a few minutes until Zach is expecting me back.

"Our lesson today has value to help you think like a Champion. The topic is Overcoming Nighttime Eating," he says.

"This topic is certainly something I need some advice on," I say. "Even after a pristine day of eating, I sometimes cave to eating out of my pantry at ten p.m." Such insanity, I admit. Surely the Genie is sick of my less-than-perfect behaviors.

"Your struggle is like that of many women," he says. "Most women have more Willpower Points in the earlier part of their day. They are more rested, and the accumulated stresses of the day have not begun to pile up. Therefore, I have found that the temptation to eat when a woman is not hungry is stronger between the hours of three in the afternoon and bedtime."

I love when I am in the normal slew of women and not an insane crazy.

"Therefore, I advise women to do something very logical but nevertheless often overlooked," he says. "Women should try to use extreme austerity in their eating in the earlier part of the day. Willpower Points are high, and women can more easily wait until they are truly hungry to eat *as well as* they can try to eat mainly vegetables and a little protein, saving some of the tastier food and calories for later in the day when Willpower Points are lower."

I like tasty food all day long.

"We all know we send kids to school in the morning, when they feel up and good. No one wants to try to corral children when they are tired or spent at night. Apply this truth to adults as well. Morning is a productive time, and humans do not need much food then. They are working and learning. However, as you well know, Willpower Points for choosing correctly begin to dwindle in the late afternoon because you are tired and spent. So be smart. Eat austerely during the day, and save your major calories and tastier food for night. Of course you need to eat some protein, good fats, and vegetables for fuel if you get truly physically hungry, but have a nose-to-the-grindstone mentality earlier in the day. Wait until you are physically hungry and then eat eggs, veggies, soups, salads, or a protein shake. When night comes and your Willpower Points are low, then you can have a little more of a treat. For example, maybe you will eat a Genie Chicken Enchilada. This is such a wise way to live life, *constantly implementing delayed gratification.* Especially since you know that Nighttime Eating is a recurring problem for you, strategize with this effort and forethought. This is how your Sane Adult knows how to live, putting Demanding Child in the playpen."

For working hard during the day, I like to reward myself at night with food. I need to reread List Six: "Pleasures and Comforts in Life besides Food."

"This is review, Young Jackie, but another important strategy to combat Nighttime Eating is to be sure your Quart Bags are accessible, that you have good food planned and prepped for dinner, as well as having yummy drinks available to drink after dinner. But as you know, this information is useless until you have ditched sugars and simple starches. Cravings are nearly impossible to resist, and they do not leave until you have consistently gotten most of the sugar and starches out of your diet."

"Cravings are no longer a problem, Genie, but I still find myself wanting something tasty at night to eat."

"Since you know that Nighttime Eating is a recurring issue for you," he says, "rereading your Ruby Journal around three in the afternoon is again a good strategy as it bathes your mind with the right thought, helping you prepare for the ensuing skirmish. On List Five in your Ruby Journal, 'Repeated Schemes My Demanding Child Uses,' be sure and list that your Demanding Child wants comfort and stimulation at night because she is tired, so you can be forewarned and mentally prepared."

The value of my Ruby Journal is inestimable. Recently, I have been carrying it around in my oversized Calvin Klein purse, so I can read it on break at work. My Demanding Child refuses to die, but reading my Ruby Journal is the best way I have found to alert and reinforce my Sane Child thinking.

He disappears, but lying on the passenger seat is a recipe with a note attached saying there is a batch of Genie Chicken Enchiladas in my fridge at home. Just having some tasty dinner to look forward to is great. I will eat austerely until dinner, paying careful attention to my hunger. The Genie is correct that my Willpower Points are up much more in the early part of the day. And I like the idea of delaying my gratification and then getting a small reward of some tasty food later in the day.

Arriving back at the office, I text Zach and he comes out to the car. The ride to the hospital is uneventful while Zach lists the main arguments he wants me to write about in the upcoming brief.

Inside the hospital, Zach and I take the elevator up to the ninth floor to meet with Mrs. Arnwine. She was in a rear-end collision and suffered a herniated disc in her neck along with a concussion. Zach is respectful beyond belief, giving her and her husband advice in all areas, even ones that do not pertain to law.

After Zach has discussed all of Mrs. Arnwine's injuries, she wiggles around in her Philadelphia collar to look at me. She asks Zach, "Who is this lovely thing?"

Zach introduces me as the "best assistant any lawyer could have" but who he will eventually "lose because she is going to law school." Zach does not know I am losing interest in going to law school.

Mrs. Arnwine becomes quite interested in the two of us. "Neither of you has a ring on. You would make a nice couple," she says.

The room has a moment of tension, and Zach does not respond. The silence is upsetting, so I decide to speak, "What a nice thing to say, Mrs. Arnwine, but Zach has a girlfriend."

"Well," she says, "she could not be as pretty as you."

Trying to get past the moment. Zach jumps in, "Mr. Arnwine, did anyone happen to get pictures of the damaged vehicle?" Good one, Zach.

However, Mrs. Arnwine will not let Zach go in that direction. Her pain meds are giving her a lot of chutzpah. "I would consider dropping that other girl if I were you, Mr. Boltz. Why, this girl is as pretty as a movie star. And look how she stares at you so adoringly. She is crazy about you."

Oh, heavens. Is this some kind of fortune teller? Or is she just an old woman on heavy meds that wants to air her opinions? How could this be happening to me?

"I am good at reading women, Mr. Boltz, and your assistant is infatuated with you," she continues.

Zach stands up to leave. "You rest, Mrs. Arnwine, and I will call you to-morrow." We all shake hands, and Zach and I leave.

Walking down the hall to the elevator, my stomach feels upset again like it did at the Titans game. When we reach the elevator, Zach breaks the silence. "She must have been on some heavy drugs," Zach offers.

Feeling terribly uncomfortable, I don't know how to move on. Gosh, the elevator is taking a long time. We stand there in silence, both looking at the elevator sign, watching to see when it will arrive.

Finally, I speak. "That was embarrassing to me."

"I am sure it was," he says. "But I know she is just an old woman on high pain meds. Don't let it bother you."

Zach turns to look at me, and I look back. His smooth olive skin, his thick brown hair, his strong eyebrows, and that white starched shirt all combine together to make me feel like I might fall down. I frantically search for something clever to say while he is looking at me, but I cannot think of one single thing.

The elevator is still not here. "Want to grab lunch on the way back to the office?" he asks. "We have not finished discussing the brief."

I have written many briefs and, in my opinion, we are through outlining it, but lunch sounds great to me.

"Okay," I say, trying to be very casual. My stomach is still in knots, but I am physically hungry, and I would like to eat.

Stopping at the Rolf and Daughters restaurant, we are seated, and Zach talks about a couple of issues we have already gone over on the way to the hospital. We order and while we are waiting on our food, Zach blurts out, "Jack, I have been doing what you said, trying to overlook issues with Rachel, to accept her, and I think I am making progress. To be honest, I did not know couples were supposed to have so many problems in their relationships. I am trying to overlook a lot of our differences. One big problem we face is where we should go to church. She has agreed to visit a couple churches that I have recommended. However, the only church she is truly interested in attending is the one she grew up in."

I know what church he is talking about. It is where the blue bloods go. Actually, it is a great church with a lot of concern for the poor.

"I like her parents' church," Zach says, "but it is not me. I would rather go to a more casual environment."

I understand this problem with finding the right church. I struggled with it for the first year I was in Nashville.

"I want to visit your church," he says. "I have heard positive things about it."

The thought of seeing Rachel every Sunday morning is not very positive to me.

"But Rachel is not interested?" I ask.

"No, she is not," he says, and he looks down at the table.

There is quite a silence, and a man I do not know who is from my parents' generation walks up to the table. In my opinion, Zach is visibly upset by the man's presence. Jumping to his feet, Zach extends his hand to the man. "Mr. Hanover, nice to see you," Zach is quick to say. Mr. Hanover? So this is Rachel's Chick-Fil-A father.

"Yes, hello there, Zach," he says as his eyes flash to me.

"Let me introduce my legal assistant, Jackie. Jackie and I have just been to the hospital to pick up a new case."

Zach feels the need to explain to his future father-in-law that I'm not anything to worry about, simply a legal assistant. Mr. Hanover is not impressed with Zach's description of me. In fact, he seems a little upset that Zach is lunching with a female. I laugh to myself as I think how innocuous I am. I want to say, *I am just fat Jackie. No worries about me replacing your blue-blood daughter, Mr. Hanover.*

"Rachel said she is playing doubles in the Nashville tennis tournament this week," her dad continues.

"Yes, sir," Zach says. "She and her partner should do well."

I guess Mr. Hanover just wanted to bring up his daughter's name, to see how Zach responded in front of me. This is all kind of bizarre.

Mr. Hanover looks at me again, with disdain, as if I am a hooligan. He looks back at Zach and says, "I will see you at dinner tonight, Zach?"

"Yes, sir. See you then," Zach says, still standing.

The persona of Mr. Hanover is strong. I have heard he is a millionaire many times. There was definitely tension in that whole conversation. Mr. Hanover leaves, and Zach is visibly agitated.

"What was going on there?" I ask.

"He did not like me having lunch with you, Jack," he explains.

Me? I think. *Fat ole me?* Like I am a threat to skinny, high-class Rachel? Ridiculous.

"Well, that is crazy," I say.

Zach looks up at me, and his eyes stare into mine. We get the check and go back to the office to grind out the afternoon's work.

Lesson 14

Handling Social Situations Like a Champion

Friday, October 31   Weight: 151   Pounds lost: 24   Still to lose: 21

Tonight is Eva's Halloween party. Because I am going as a nightclub singer, I bought a black wig to wear that is teased out to the atmosphere along with a floor-length silky red dress. I decide to wear huge fake eyelashes and carry around a microphone. Detesting these kinds of events, I have to pretend to be excited about them.

My text message beeps, and it is Brad, the nice guy that sat by me in the singles' zone at church last Sunday. He is a doctor and is doing research with stem cells. Although his glasses are outdated and his plaid shirt is wrinkled, he gets a pass for his work ethic as a doctor.

This is Brad Chockley, remember me? I sat by you in church last Sunday. I got your number from our mutual friend, Heather. Are you going to the same service this Sunday? Would you like to go to lunch afterward?

What do I have to lose? Maybe the guy is amazing and is my soul mate. I laugh at my own optimism, knowing that it would be a miracle if this non-fashionable brainy guy were my soul mate. I text back and accept. At least, he knows my still-large size and must be okay with it.

After work, I drive home and get dressed for the party. Honestly, I feel pretty good. I can certainly tell I am down twenty-four pounds, and this red dress is slimming.

Driving to Eva's, I try to be late on purpose. Beth and Richard are always late, and I want there to be someone I am comfortable talking to before I arrive. Also, I hate navigating the food at these events. There is rarely anything available to eat on my program, and I end up eating some of the Trash Food that is served.

Not surprisingly, the Genie appears in my front passenger seat.

"Today's lesson is Handling Social Situations like a Champion," he says. "This short lesson will prepare your mind before the Halloween party."

Knowing there will probably not be good food for me at this event has already stirred up a few feelings of discouragement. And of course, there is the added uncomfortableness of seeing the dreaded skinnies, Rachel and Eva.

"During most social situations," he says, "you have to assume there will probably *not* be good food choices available for you. Social events are well known to have a plethora of sugary and refined carb foods because that is what most people like. Occasionally, you will find some available good protein choices, raw veggies, salads, fruit, and food that you can eat, but more often not. Instead of feeling deprived at such an event, feel happy that you have been given the secrets to escape Trash Food. Actually, many of my past *Skinny School* clients learn to feel sorry for the people at the event who are still trapped in the Food Dungeon scenario. They rejoice in their feelings of self-mastery and their newly acquired knowledge. My *Skinny School* students do not feel self-pity over missing a three-minute taste experience because they are going after something much more satisfying, thinness."

In the past, that thinking has certainly not been my go-to thinking at these events.

"At social events, my *Skinny School* students try to find good food choices, of course, but if they are not available, then they do not partake of the Trash Food. Being prepared, my Champion students always carry a nut mixture or an apple in their purses. Or sometimes they stash a small bag of raw veggies and a couple pieces of cheese somewhere. They do not bring these out at the party, as that would be rude, but eat it shortly after the party. There are ways to overcome most situations if some forethought is taken."

This behavior seems extreme to me, but of course Champions think like that. They do whatever it takes to reach their goals.

As I arrive at Eva's apartment, the Genie disappears, and on the passenger seat is a small Ziploc bag of nuts along with a small bag of string cheese, which I slip into my purse.

Walking into Eva's apartment, I see that there are forty or fifty hilariously dressed people. Rachel is dressed as a cave woman and Zach as a cave man. If there are prizes, they should win first place. Luckily they are across the room, so I do not have to speak to them yet. Eva is dressed as a monkey, with brown tights, a brown leotard, a tail, and a little hat. She looks tinier than ever. Beth and Richard are dressed in Renaissance clothes, with Beth being the princess and Richard the squire. Making my way over to the food table, I survey the contents to see if there is any food I can eat. Not surprisingly, it is full of chips, M&M's, sugar cookies resembling pumpkins, and brownies. The Genie said to expect this.

Turning down the loud music, Eva announces to everyone to get a partner of the opposite sex because we are going to play a version of couples *Family Feud*. I hate these moments when everyone is told to get a partner. Glancing around, I notice everyone is pairing up but me. I look at this one guy, but he glances away. Obviously, he does not want to be paired up with a chubby nightclub singer. All my earlier feelings of looking good in this red dress evaporate. The desperation starts to set in as everyone is paired up. Eva yells, "Did everyone get a partner?"

Terrified that everyone will realize no one wanted to be paired with me, I do not say anything but slip into the kitchen and try to look busy.

"Okay, let's begin," Eva says, totally unaware that I am still unpaired. The crowd laughs and roars at each other's funny answers in the den, and there I am in the kitchen, bustling around like Snow White, as though housekeeping was my calling and passion.

"What are you doing in here?" asks a familiar voice that at once I recognize as Zach's.

"Cleaning up a bit," I say, as if I am totally happy to be the household help.

"You should be in this game," he says. "This is the kind of game at which you are amazing. Rachel and I got out the first round."

Well, I would have liked to have been in the game too, I think, but do not let on and instead laugh in a fake way. "Maybe I will play the next round," I say, trying to sound like I am in a good mood when what I really want is to drive through Wendy's and get the works.

Rachel walks in the kitchen. "Jackie! What a cute outfit!" she says, as she pours herself a diet drink. Her cave woman outfit shows off her million-dollar legs and her twenty-three-inch waist. Who wouldn't want to date this gorgeous piece of prehistoric meat?

Rachel starts picking at Zach. "Zach, why did you say 'Bring them books'? That was a terrible answer, Zach."

Zach looks at me as he knows I have no idea what she is talking about. He explains for my benefit: "The question in the game was, 'Name something you would do for a friend if they were sick at home with a bad cold.'"

Rachel jumps in, "'Bring them lunch.' 'Bring them flowers.' Those are good answers. But 'Bring them books'? Ha-ha, that was a terrible answer, Zach."

Rachel is teasing, but I can tell Zach does not like his answer being criticized.

"I would like a good book if I was sick," I say. "A good book can get me out of a funk faster than anything." Of course, I am a book freak.

Zach looks at me in a pleased way, but Rachel does not stop. "A good book? That is the last thing I want when I am down. Bring me a new pair of diamond earrings! Now, there is a good answer!" She laughs as if she has given the best answer in the universe.

Zach glances at me and smiles just a tad. I guess he thinks she is adorable. In my opinion, she is a shallow cave woman.

For the next game, the group plays Catch Phrase. Circling the room, we count off one through four to make the teams. Even chubs get to play this time.

Secretly I glance at my watch, counting down how much longer until I can excuse myself without looking needy or upset. Chubby girls have learned all the tricks in knowing how to leave parties early.

Catch Phrase is over. After quietly saying good-bye to Beth, I slip out the door. The temptation to medicate my emotions with some fast-food drive-through appears. But I know that what I really want is to look as skinny as the cave woman and monkey just looked. Fortunately, I read my Ruby Journal before the Halloween party, knowing that these kind of social events can upset me. Having my brain bathed with Ruby Journal thoughts—such as how upset I will be in the morning if I cave in to my Demanding Child right now—I gulp down the contents of the little bags that the Genie gave me and speed home to get my Quart Bags, take a bath, get some tasty hot herbal tea, and get lost in a novel. My Demanding Child wants some self-soothing, and I will give it to her, just not with Trash Food!

Lesson 15

How to Eat in Restaurants

Like A Champion

Sunday, November 9   Weight: 148   Pounds lost: 27   Still to lose: 18

Today is the day that Zach and I leave for Boca Raton at 4:00 p.m. I cannot think about that now, though, because I am supposed to meet non-*GQ* Brad at church. He already texted me to ask where I plan to sit. He seems nice enough, I guess. At least Brad seems to be a person of sincere faith, which is who I am at my core. I will not make that mistake again, like I did with Robert.

Meeting Brad at the designated seats, I immediately notice his wrinkly and baggy corduroy pants. He begins to talk about his work in stem cell research, which I can tell he is passionate about. I like a man who is passionate about his work. Obviously, this is why he does not have more time to pay attention to his grooming.

Since the service is starting, I reach for my phone to turn off the sound. There is a text from Zach. **Rachel agreed to try your church. Any seats by you?**

I text back: **Actually, there are two empty seats right here. We are near the front in the section on the left.**

In thirty seconds, Zach and Rachel are coming up the aisle, looking for me.

"A new man, Jackie?" Rachel whispers as she passes in front of me to get to her seat, just like we are best friends.

My first thought is that when she finds out he is a doctor, she will be impressed. Maybe she will think I am in her league if I marry a doctor.

After the service, Brad and Zach seem to do well together. Finding out that Zach is my boss, Brad asks, "Jackie and I are going to lunch. Would you two like to join us?"

"Oh, we would love to," Rachel interjects, "but we are having lunch with my parents at the country club."

"We are?" Zach asks, surprised. "You did not say anything about it to me."

She looks him squarely in the eye and says, "Oh, sorry. I must have forgotten."

Something is rotten in the state of Denmark—I mean, Tennessee.

Brad and I eat at McAlister's, and Brad starts a conversation again about his stem cell research. My, he is really into this stem cell stuff. His one-track mind is unattractive to me, but no one is perfect. Maybe he will grow on me. By looking at his hands, I can tell he bites his fingernails. Maybe that is what genius doctors do when they are thinking brilliant thoughts.

Getting home after lunch, I quickly finish packing, as it is almost time for Zach to pick me up to go to the airport. My heart is actually beating so strongly I can feel it.

Last week I shopped until I dropped, getting four great outfits that I feel good in. I feel a little bad about spending so much money on new clothes, but honestly, nothing in my closet fits anymore, so I give myself a pass. Right now I am wearing a yellow wool jacket with black pencil-leg trousers and the best-looking Coach boots and purse I could find. Maybe I am still eighteen pounds overweight, but being twenty-seven pounds down is invigorating.

Turning around, I see the Genie putting my last odds and ends into my suitcase. The Genie is adding a new turquoise blouse with rhinestone buttons that looks like silk but is probably an imitation. "What is that?" I ask.

"Just a little present for you to wear on your trip," he says. In my opinion, it is too dressy to wear on a business trip, but I let him pack it. I do look good in turquoise.

"Today the topic is How to Eat in Restaurants like a Champion," he begins. "As you know, the success of a *Skinny School* student lies in how she thinks. That is why we are going over every small nuance of your life, so you will have the right strategy in how to think about almost every situation."

I wonder if I will ever completely embrace this Champion mind-set.

"Restaurants present a big temptation to women as they offer the experience of *new*. Humans love newness, and they feel deprived if they think they are going to miss out on a new experience."

He is right. Seeing new food concoctions, I want to experience them.

"Actually, it is normal and healthy to desire variety," he says. "And there are many new food experiences for you in the realm of proteins, vegetables, and good fats. As I have said before, you do not have to go outside the Creator's infinite choices of great foods to find food that is good for you as well as delicious. However, restaurants offer temptation in that they also offer new experiences in foods that are *not* good for you. This is what we will discuss today."

Whenever I walk into a restaurant, the yummy Trash Foods start whispering my name.

"Do not tell yourself you are not allowed new taste experiences," he says. "You are! You are only not allowed new Trash Food experiences. It is wonderful to try new fish that is cooked in legitimate ways, to order vegetables cooked with new seasoning, or to taste new salads. Do not fall for the lie that you do not get to continue to try new taste experiences. Eating great food does not have to be boring, but being thin does demand that you keep yourself away from Trash Food. There can be no self-pity here. Remember, the pleasures in life are infinite, and you have to constantly refer to your Ruby Journal to remind yourself of what pleasures you like, such as those you have recorded on List Six. Your Demanding Child will forever continue to suggest reasons why you should eat Trash Food. Eventually, your mind will be so strongly trained, though, that you will be able to talk her out of her pleas. But until then, your Ruby Journal must be repeatedly read."

This lesson sounds like review to me.

"Also, I want to warn you about the large portions at restaurants," he says. "Even if the food is healthy, restaurants often serve ridiculously oversized portions, as they know this delights the Demanding Child in their customers. Get in the habit of only eating half or two-thirds of your meal and asking for a take-out box. Divide your food mentally on your plate as soon as it arrives, telling yourself what you will eat and what you will take home."

That is hard to do when the food is so yummy.

"Another strategy to use in restaurants is to fill up on zero-calorie drinks," he says. "You can order water with lemon, iced tea, herbal tea, coffee, and many other delicious drinks. These good drinks make you feel less deprived."

I often don't order decaf coffee after dinner to save the money, even though I would enjoy it. But if I'm not eating dessert, then I can afford it, right?

"Restaurant behavior must be practiced," he says. "The temptation will always be great, as new taste experiences are extremely compelling to humans. But with training your mind, you can handle any restaurant in any situation. However, when you do experience some failure, be sure you do not succumb to Hog-Wild Mentality and instead record the pothole in your Ruby Journal so you can avoid it next time."

Try, fail, record, evaluate, try again. He will not let up. But actually, that is good. I need someone barking at me to *get* on the bus and *stay* on the bus because my Demanding Child still wants to leap out the window.

"Just remember, there is no situation that you cannot outsmart eventually if you will do the work to dissect your failure, frequently read your Ruby Journal, and *get immediately right back on the bus when you fall off.* I packed some nuts, apples, and peanut butter in your suitcase. I am going to get a massage in Bangladesh, so I will see you soon," he says, as he disintegrates.

Hearing Zach's car pull up, I walk outside with my suitcase. My scarf is deep yellow, rust, and black, and it is exquisite. Zach does a long stare when he sees me approaching his car with my suitcase. "Jack! You look great," he says. It is a compliment you might give your sister, I know, but I deposit the compliment into my soul for safekeeping.

"Thanks," I casually say, trying to hide my delight.

Before we are barely out of the parking lot, Zach asks, "How long have you been dating Brad?"

Shocked by the nonbusiness subject so soon, I reply, "I am not dating him. We have just sat together in church a couple of times, and he asked me to lunch."

"He seems like an easy kind of guy to have around," Zach says.

"He is great company if you like talking about stem cells," I say and laugh. Zach smiles and drops the subject—and so do I. As I hear myself say that, I know that the kick is not there for me as far as Brad. However, I will not cut the strings quite yet because he is a nice guy, and again, maybe he is the best I can do.

After our uneventful plane ride, we grab a quick dinner at the hotel restaurant, going over every possible angle we can think of that might help us with the deposition in the morning. I only eat two-thirds of my meal. I get to a five in fullness and have the willpower to stop. The Genie would be proud.

"I will see you in the morning in the lobby at seven for breakfast. Is that okay?" Zach asks.

"Sure," I smile. At 4:00 a.m. At 2:00 a.m. Whenever you say, Zach.

"The depositions start at nine. If we can finish by five or so, I would like to go to Seasons 52 restaurant," he says in a perfect business tone.

"Do you want me to make reservations, just in case we can make it?" I ask.

"I already did, for seven thirty" he says.

Zach already made reservations at 52 Seasons for the two of us? Somehow, someway, I will see that this deposition runs like clockwork, so we are free to make that reservation time.

Zach is brilliant, as usual, during the deposition, and I did not do too badly either, although I would never say that out loud to anyone. At one point, I slip Zach a note to mention the doctor's visit during which the man in question (on the other side) said something that he contradicted today. I can tell by Zach's face that he appreciates it. The deposition is now over early, and we head back to the hotel in the rental car.

"Zach, that was the best deposition I have ever witnessed, and I used to go to them all the time when I worked for Fortwright. The way you built the case, step by step, was spectacular. And I loved the way you cornered the defendant into admitting that he might be confused about the facts. It was nothing short of brilliant."

That was some pretty heavy praise, but it is all true. Zach is a phenomenal lawyer, as good as they come. Every word I said was true.

That grin that is usually kept in check starts to show. "You liked it?"

He wants to talk some more about the deposition, I can tell, so I go through the whole two hours, summarizing what he did right, what I liked, what was really smart and savvy. He listens and eats it up, like we are watching highlight films of a quarterback making successive successful touchdown passes. His performance today was stellar, so critiquing it is easy for me.

We arrive back at the hotel at 5:30 p.m., and Zach asks if we can meet downstairs in the lobby at 7:00 p.m. "It is a dressy restaurant," he says.

"Okay," I say. The turquoise top that the Genie packed for me might be the perfect thing. I know Zach has a girlfriend, but regardless, I get myself ready to dine with a prince.

I enter the lobby at 7:02, and Zach is already there. I have swept my hair up into a French knot but left many strands falling down. My pearls are small and soft, and I feel I look better than I have in years. Maybe not smokin' skinny yet, but wow, what an improvement. Zach smiles as I approach and watches me. Maybe I am making this up, but he seems to communicate approval.

"That is a great color for you, Jack," he says as we walk toward the parking lot. Zach has a tie on, which surprises me. I love ties on men. Ties speak of order, restraint, power, and class...all adjectives that describe Zach.

Arriving at Seasons 52 restaurant, we find that our table is ready, and we are seated. I love these places with white tablecloths, three waiters per table, and lots of low lights and dark wood. Zach has a girlfriend, I remind myself. This is only a business dinner because we have to travel together.

We both order spiced ice tea and split an appetizer of stuffed mushrooms. Zach orders the rib eye, and I order grilled wild-caught tilapia. I am counting carbs and sugar secretly in my mind. Our Caesar salads are brought, and Zach's expression changes.

"Jack, here is what I want to talk about tonight," he says.

Okay, I think. The Torrey case. The Whiteson case. The Pomanic case. Fine. Whatever he wants to talk about, I am game. I think about how this turquoise top showcases my shoulders and neckline, some of my best features. I hope Zach notices.

"I need some advice, and you seem to be the person who gives me the best advice," Zach starts.

Maybe he wants to talk about the deposition today some more. That is fine with me. I sure do like my hair in this French knot. I am glad I brought all those bobby pins so I could do it up tonight.

"I need some advice again on Rachel," he says, not looking at me.

Rachel? Gulp. We are going to talk about that unpleasant topic? The delight of the night is whisked away, much as the light disappears when you blow out a candle. Rachel, little size zero, snotty Rachel. I can't think of anything I would rather *not* talk about. Last time when he wanted advice on Rachel, I helped him move toward her. I don't know if I can be that generous again.

"What is going on?" I ask, disappointed that this is our topic.

"I hope you will keep this in strict confidence," he says. "I thought about talking to my father about this, and I still might do that, but for some reason, I want to know your opinion. You seem to get people so well. I am not even sure how to explain this, but…well…do you think it is normal to feel a little bored with someone you are seriously dating? I understand that women care a lot about makeup, clothes, and subjects that men are not interested in, but how much is okay? Honestly, I feel bored with many of Rachel's topics. I feel like I should be a better listener and more interested in her subjects."

"Actually," I say, "my sister Jessica has been studying marriage, and she told me that part of love is learning to be interested in someone else's topics," I begrudgingly say, knowing that this, again, is giving Rachel slack and grace.

"Your sister is married," he says, "so of course the rules are different after you have made a lifelong commitment. But Rachel and I are not married, and I am trying to decide if a couple should have more in common than we do."

The temptation to throw out my personal opinion, that Rachel is a skank and not worthy to untie his shoe laces, is quickly dismissed. I think hard, and instead of dissing Rachel like I would like to, I try to be helpful.

I say, "My grandmother used to say, 'Do not marry someone you can live with, but marry someone you can't live without.' She said that when the winds and storms of life come in the marriage, which they will, you will always know you are with the right person."

When I quote my grandmother's advice, Zach's eyeballs get almost as large as the broccoli crowns on my plate. They lock with mine. Those eye locks with Zach feel as rich and deep as if I have been given the keys to the royal treasury of the universe. What is it about a man like Zach that is so griping, so powerful, so consuming? I feel completely lost in those four seconds, and at the same time, I feel completely found. The eye lock makes me want to cry and laugh, both at the same time.

Zach speaks. "Marry someone you can't live without? Jack, that is a huge thought."

Here I go again, giving Zach the fuel and motivation to move toward Rachel. He knows he cannot live without her, even though they have issues. I gave him the key so he would be able to make that last jump over the hurdle, and now he can propose. I cannot believe how I do this. I want to lie down and sleep for two years. When I wake up, I can heal from the nightmare of Zach's upcoming engagement.

Zach's eyes dance. They explode with fire. I just helped him over the fence. I just gave him the thought he needed so he could quit dillydallying around. The fireworks going off in his eyes now tell me that he has given himself freedom to propose. Even though she has some chick topics that bore him, he realizes he can't live without her, and this is just one of the little things about Rachel he will have to learn to accept. To the degree that Zach seems elated with his new insight and freedom, I feel bummed and spent.

We eat the rest of our dinner, discussing only the deposition of the day. I can't wait to get back to the hotel and go to bed, getting rid of this horrible, terrible, no good, very bad day. The proposal is coming.

Lesson 16

Handling Holidays Like a Champion

Wednesday, November 26   *Weight: 145*   *Pounds lost: 23*   *Still to lose: 15*

Today is the Wednesday before Thanksgiving. I am driving to Memphis early in the morning to eat Thanksgiving dinner with my sisters and their families. Having never been through a Thanksgiving meal with my new, enlightened Genie thinking, I wonder how I will fare facing the pumpkin pie.

Eva, our self-imposed office social chairman, has put together an ice skating event tonight with the young people in the office. She has invited Richard and Beth, Zach and Rachel, me (and I invited wardrobe-deficient Brad), and her new boyfriend, Chad. Her new hunk, Chad, is a bodybuilder. The first time I met Chad, he told me how his coach wants him to eat six thousand calories a day so he can bulk up for competitions. Oh, dear.

The troops are arriving at the skating rink. Brad, with his saggy jeans and faded sweatshirt, engages Zach in what appears to be a deep conversation. Getting wind of the conversation, I can tell Brad is talking about stem cells again. Does he not have another topic?

Everyone is getting on their skates, even Bodybuilder Man, Chad. Chad just bought a new Canon camera, and he is taking pictures of everyone. Chubby people do not particularly like people taking random shots of them. Chubs like me like to get behind someone and just smile pretty. However, I am curious about Chad's camera and ask him if I can look at it. Someday, I would like one of these.

Rachel looks like an ad for Patagonia for what one is supposed to wear while ice skating. She really is a cutie pie. A mean cutie pie.

Zach says he does not skate, and actually I have sore muscles from my DVD workout, so I sit out too. Brad and Rachel are both good skaters and are having fun zooming around the ice, leaving Zach and me alone to drink hot tea. The ice skating rink is already decorated for Christmas, and the piped music is the familiar "Chestnuts roasting on an open fire…"

"How are things going for you, Jack?" Zach asks. I love this about Zach, asking questions to engage others. He is the best at this. And he is not a phony; he really cares about other people.

"I guess, okay," I say. Dating Brad is certainly not working out, I think, but I do not want to discuss my dating life with Zach.

"Are things hard for you now?" he asks.

Surprised by the question, I am even more surprised by my honest answer, "Yes, there are some things I would like to change."

"Like what?" he asks.

The music is now, "I'll…be home…for Christmas…"

The shield is coming off my heart. I decide to tell him *most* of the truth. "I still want to lose these last fifteen pounds," I say. "And I want to figure out my life calling as far as work because I am not sure it is law school anymore. I would really like to write novels, but I do not know how to do that and support myself."

I do, however, have the sense to *not* tell him that I am ready to meet and marry my life partner…somebody *exactly like him.*

"What about you, Zach? Anything you would like to change?" This bold question seems legitimate to ask in light of the fact that he just asked me the same thing. But now, thinking about it, I am embarrassed I asked that. Of course, there is nothing he wants to change. He is getting ready to marry Rachel, be a top Nashville lawyer, and have little Zachites running around with pacifiers and American Girl dolls in their arms.

"Well, sometimes I feel lonely," Zach says, looking down. "Not that I need more people around. It is more of a *depth* I wish I felt…"

I sit quietly and wait to see if he is going to say more.

"Funny, but there are a few moments when I do not feel lonely, I have noticed," he continues. "These moments surprise me." His eyes rise to meet mine, and they almost burn because of the intensity. With that, he gets up to walk to the rail to look at the skaters. I guess the "few moments" he is referring to are those moments he and Rachel share intense conversations. I am not sure. Maybe I just pushed him again to hurry and propose, so he will be lonely less often.

"Oh, the weather outside is frightful, but the fire is so delightful…" the music continues.

Hearing Zach say he is sometimes lonely makes me remember how much of my life I have felt lonely. Although I notice I am *not* lonely when Zach is around. That is when I feel happy. Knowing that his engagement is on the horizon, maybe I should consider moving back to Memphis with my sisters in order to avoid having to see him all the time. Maybe I could begin to heal and get over him. I will talk to my sisters about it tomorrow when I see them for Thanksgiving dinner.

The others return from skating, and Eva recommends that we all go to Jimmy Kelly's Steakhouse to eat, but Beth and Richard say they need to relieve their babysitter, and Rachel says she already has other plans. My excuse to leave is that I need to get up early to drive to Memphis. Luckily, the whole group dissolves. Brad says he will call me tomorrow, and I say okay, but I know it is just a matter of finding the right time to tell him that we can only be friends.

Snowflakes are beginning to fall. The beauty of the snowflakes and the barrenness of my soul make a strong contrast. My jolly Middle Eastern friend appears on my passenger seat.

"Hello, Young Jackie," the Genie says. Maybe it is good he shows up because I feel my Demanding Child wanting to medicate my self-pity over my stinking life.

"Tonight we are going to talk about Handling Holidays like a Champion," he says.

Ugh. Holidays. The horrible food season. I gain weight over the holidays every year.

"Incredible temptation is coming, and if you are not overprepared, you will cave in to all the abundance of Trash Food," he begins. "During the holidays, there are, as you know, numerous social events at which an abundance of Trash Food temptation is thrown at you."

Pumpkin pie. Apple pie. Blueberry pie.

"The secret of coasting through the holidays is to overbathe your mind with correct thought," he explains. "Expect the Trash Food to come. When you see it, be ready to say to yourself, 'This is what I knew was coming, and I am glad I have prepared my mind.' Being prepared mentally is everything in these social situations with Trash Food."

Nostalgia hits me and a certain sadness descends upon me. "Genie, growing up, we had cookie bakes and long afternoons in the kitchen where my mom, sisters, and I made fudge, banana-nut bread for neighbors, and every holiday delight you can imagine. Having so many fond memories with food during the holidays, I somehow now feel cheated not getting to enjoy all that food."

Ready for a rebuke from the Genie, I brace myself. However, his eyes are tender, which is a surprise. Usually, he is somewhat harsh in responding to my obvious self-pity.

"I understand all the love and memories that are associated with the holidays and food," he says kindly. "However, now is the time to create new traditions to celebrate the holidays besides Trash Food. Now is the time to create healthy food choices along with other activities that joyfully celebrate the holidays. You do not have to miss the celebration just because you do not have Trash Food."

"What other activities and traditions?" I ask. Holidays scream Trash Food to me.

"New traditions could be games or activities," he says. "Volunteering, going to holiday shows, making bonfires, or doing puzzles together are just a few ideas. Food that is healthy must be planned and prepped. There is no reason to fall into eating Trash Food just because it is a holiday. Do you see how ludicrous that is? Is it not ridiculous to eat Trash Food and then be upset over your weight gain? How much better to eat healthy food and celebrate the holidays in other ways. Maybe you can start new traditions such as hiking, buying toys for needy children, or even just going to movies. The list of ways to celebrate the holidays is endless. Your Demanding Child wants the pleasure of Trash Food, but you must corral her and find other stimulation during the holidays. This is obviously work to create new traditions. However, at the end of the season, you will have *not* gained weight and will still have great memories. Holidays are about family and spiritual meaning. They are not about Trash Food."

Celebrating the holidays without Trash Food will take mega effort. I associate the whole season with Trash Food. And I hate puzzles.

"Champions know there is a great daily resistance in achieving their goals," he says, "so they put in extra effort during rough times. Yes, you will *experience some discomfort,* but it is tolerable because you have something you really want: thinness. Repeatedly you must realize that experiencing taste sensations is *not* in your current Top Four Life Goals. You also know that you have to sometimes give up *good* to get the *best,* so no self-pity! No deprivation! Only excitement about having a plan out of your prior dungeon of chubbiness."

It is amazing to me how the Genie gives me these talks, and I feel empowered. But then his talks lose ground in my mind, and I want to revert to saying yes to my Demanding Child's requests. Repeatedly bathing my mind with my Ruby Journal is necessary because I so quickly return to what is comfortable and easy.

"Handling Trash Food during the holidays is one of the hardest lessons in *Skinny School.* The memories and delight associated with childhood and holidays are difficult to overcome. But you are not the norm. You are now a Champion thinker. You are no longer in the dark about all the schemes of your Demanding Child. The veil has been ripped, and you see clearly."

I admit my understanding has been somewhat widened. However, I am not the Champion thinker he is describing. My hope is that if I continue to bathe my mind in *Skinny School* thought, I might somehow, someway, someday eventually think like a Champion.

"I have left you a recipe of Genie Chicken Divan in your refrigerator at your apartment," he says and then disintegrates. I am not sure why, but

I feel very emotional. Maybe it is a combination of the beautiful snow, the Christmas music I just heard, and the thoughts of my childhood, cooking in the kitchen with my now deceased mother, but nevertheless, I start sobbing. And I cannot stop. Even though I have much to be grateful for, the holidays are the worst for single people. Brad is definitely not the right one, and I am alone, just like always. I guess it will always be like this.

The streets are slippery with the snowflakes. My car is even sliding some when I hit the brakes. Hey, that guy has a red light, but, but…

I wake up. There's a paramedic standing over me. "Who should we call, miss?"

"Beth Willibanks, six-eight-three-four-five-five-two," I say, barely able to speak.

I am semiconscious the entire ride to the hospital in the ambulance. As soon as they wheel me into the emergency room, the doctors and nurses begin hooking me up to machines, examining me, administering X-rays, and basically, taking me through the works.

When I wake up again, I am in a hospital room. Beth, Richard, Zach, and Rachel are there. Beth must have contacted Zach. "How are you?" Beth asks.

"Do you know a good personal injury lawyer I could call?" I ask, even though it is quite an effort to speak. The room laughs, knowing that obviously my mental facilities are intact with that remark.

That is, the whole room laughs except Rachel. I hear her whisper to Zach, "It's late. Can we leave now? She's okay."

I hear Zach say to her, "We are waiting on the last set of X-rays."

Into the room walks a young, cheerful doctor. "It is now five minutes after midnight, so it is officially Thanksgiving," he says. "Happy Thanksgiving, everybody." The group's energy is somewhat high, and being surrounded by friends feels encouraging.

"How is she, doc?" Zach asks. "She had better be okay by Monday because her boss does not like her missing work." Beth and Richard laugh at Zach's comment, but again, Rachel is stone faced.

"Jackie might have a slight concussion, but we are not sure yet," the doctor says. He begins to explain some tests they are still doing.

Again I see Rachel tugging on Zach's arm as she whispers, "She is going to be all right. Can we leave?" This time I cannot hear Zach's response to Rachel. The doctor makes a few more comments and then says they are going to keep me overnight to watch me closely. Beth offers to stay and says Richard will take care of Alexis, but I insist I will be okay. Beth and Richard leave. I look around for Rachel, but I don't see her; only Zach is left.

"Where is Rachel?" I ask, still being a little doped up and not having the self-control I usually have.

"Her brother came and picked her up," he says.

Again, not muzzling my mouth like I should, I asked, "Why did you not leave too?" I would normally never say that kind of bold thing to Zach. These drugs unhinge the tongue.

"Because I had to stay to check on you. If something happens to you, I have to go back to writing briefs."

I laugh, but it hurts my head. "Aren't you getting ready to propose?" Even drugged, I know it is a bad thing to say, but the drugs make me not care.

"No, Jack, I am not proposing, *not hardly,*" he says. Being woozy, I can barely keep my eyelids open, and I fall back asleep.

When I wake up, it is morning, and Zach is semilying in a recliner on the other side of the room, asleep himself. My medicine has worn off somewhat but not completely. A nurse enters with a breakfast tray and announces that my tests are all normal, and I can check out after breakfast. After I eat and get dressed, the staff puts me in a wheelchair to take me to the discharge area to get in Zach's car. Although I cannot wait to get home and go back to sleep, I make an effort at conversation.

"Happy Thanksgiving, Zach, and thank you so much for staying last night," I say. "Are you going to the Hanovers' for Thanksgiving dinner today?"

"Plans have changed," he says. Trying to stay engaged in the conversation, I force my eyelids to stay open.

"What are you talking about?" I ask, not really caring about the answer.

"Rachel wanted me to leave the hospital last night, but I told her that I wanted to make sure you were all right first. She said she did not like the way she has been treated lately and she wanted to break up. When I did not argue, she stomped off and said that she had called her brother and he was picking her up. When I did not argue with that, she said, 'We are over for good because you do not care anymore.' Again, I did not argue, and she burst into tears and ran off."

This story wakes me up somewhat. "I'm sorry," I lie.

"I texted her," Zach continues, "and told her I would come over today and we would talk. But Jack, I cannot keep doing this. I know relationships are hard, but this one is too hard."

I do not say anything. He continues. "Her father texted me already this morning and wants me to come talk to him today, too."

"Oh, boy, that will be a lot of fun," I say, thinking about how intimidating Rachel's Chick-Fil-A father was when I met him at the restaurant.

Zach raises his eyebrows to acknowledge that he agrees. "I feel I owe it to the family to give an explanation," he says. "But how do you tell a father that you simply do not love his daughter?"

Reaching my apartment, Zach walks me inside. Immediately I get into my bed, and he leaves. Even as I get semiexcited about Zach's breakup, my mood soon plummets as I realize now I have to watch Zach as he dates new girls, high-end girls—not middle-class, still-kind-of-chubby girls like me. The thought of how the wolves will pounce on him depresses me. My head hurts, and I desperately want to sleep.

Before dozing off, I hear my text message beep, and it is Brad, wanting to know when I will be back in town from Memphis so we can go out again. Briefly I text Brad back about what happened last night and then add that it is probably best if we are just friends. I click SEND and wait, but there is no reply.

Quickly I call Jessica and give her a rundown of the last twenty-four hours. At least I will not have to confront pumpkin pie today.

Lesson 17

How to Navigate Weekends

Friday, December 5   *Weight: 144*   *Pounds Lost: 31*   *Still to lose: 14*

Zach has not mentioned his breakup with Rachel, and neither have I. We have had an especially busy week, trying to close his legal files before the end of the year.

The temperature in Nashville is setting a record-breaking low. Last night the low was nine degrees, and the city is now in an uproar with a snowstorm brewing. Attorney Simpson sends the staff home early, as Nashville drivers do not have a clue about navigating icy streets. Thankfully, I make it to my apartment without an accident.

I jack up the heat and boil some water for a cup of caramel chocolate decaf herbal tea. A text message from Beth beeps.

Do you have power? We just lost ours.

I immediately call her. "Beth, come spend the night over here. As you know, I have an extra bedroom and lots of food in the fridge. Besides, I miss Alexis."

"Are you sure? We could try to get a hotel and—"

"That is insane, Beth, when I have this whole empty, warm apartment. I will start dinner. Pack up the baby and come on over," I say very convincingly.

"You are the best, Jackie," she oozes.

"I am excited we are having a slumber party," I say. "I hope Richard is game."

"He will be thrilled to not spend money on a hotel room," she laughs. As she speaks, I realize how expensive a nonworking wife and a baby must be. We hang up, and I begin to think about what task I should do first to prepare for my guests.

My text message beeps again, but this time it is from Zach.

Did your electricity go off?

I write back: No. Beth and Richard's went out, and they are spending the night over here. Did yours go out?

He writes: Yes. I am going to my parents' house.

I wish I could invite him to our slumber party, but that is just too forward. I write: Your mom is a great cook. She will take good care of you.

There is a long pause. Zach does not write back, and I am disappointed. I had hoped I would find a way to get him to come over.

Walking into the kitchen, I get out the ingredients to make Baked Orange Roughy with Cajun Seasoning. The weatherman is telling the city to bundle up, stay home, and stay warm because there are power outages all over the city, and emergency crews are working overtime.

My phone lights up again with a text from Zach.

I just talked to Richard. He says you are cooking dinner for them. Can I get an invitation too if I bring vegetables and salad? And then another text pops up: Maybe I can sleep on the sofa.

I write back: Ha-ha, I bet the grocery shelves are cleared out by now. You know how desperate Nashville gets with snow. But come. We will have a spades tournament.

See you in 45, he writes.

Forty-five minutes is not very long, and again, I am not sure what tasks to conquer first with only a few minutes to prepare. **"Would you like some help with the housework and dinner?" a friendly voice asks, and as I turn around, my whole apartment is instantly squeaky clean, and the orange roughy is prepared, ready to go into the oven.**

"Also, there are fresh sheets on the beds, and I brought in wood for the fireplace," the Genie says.

Initially feeling stressed by the upcoming night's plan, I begin to relax as I realize the work to prepare for the night is done. Gathering my Ruby Journal, I sit down, ready to take notes.

"The topic tonight is Navigating Weekends like a Champion," he begins. "Weekends have their own flavor in contrast to the work week. In human minds, there is a subconscious feeling that weekends should be relaxing and enjoyable. Not that this thought is wrong, but your Demanding Child takes this thought and tells you to apply this thought to your food consumption."

I still forget there are other ways in life to entertain myself or soothe myself *without* food.

"Plans are often made on the weekend that include eating out or going to events where food is served. The Demanding Child is waiting in the shadows to convince you that this situation is special or that you deserve a treat. Again, this may be true, but the treat does *not* need to be Trash Food. There is no reason for you to let down on the pursuit of one of your current Top Four Life Goals on the weekend. Your mind is the battleground. If you realize extra temptation is coming because your Demanding Child always wants you to go off your program, then you will be forearmed. You will hear Demanding Child say, 'You have been grinding away all week, and now you need to reward yourself.' Again, this may be true, but there are many ways to give yourself a reward besides Trash Food or eating off your program. I would like you to make List Nine in your Ruby Journal and entitle it 'Ways to Relax, Replenish, and Reward Myself besides Food.' Weekends do not need to be a downfall, but they often are because the mind and good food choices are not prepped. Prep the mind. Prep food. *Preparation* is the mantra of Champions."

This list sounds very much like List Six, but I will attempt to fill it out.

"As you know, Demanding Child has only around twenty-five schemes, not twenty-five hundred," he says. "Weekends are one of the twenty-five. Gather yourself, and prepare for the weekend by having prepped food available and by working on your list of how to relax, replenish, and reward yourself without Trash Food or eating outside your program."

The average *Skinny School* person has twenty-five schemes to overcome, but I think my shrewd Demanding Child has 125.

"In our future lesson on Planned Cheating," he says, "we will discuss how many *Skinny School* graduates use the weekends to enjoy their Planned Cheating, but that is not until they reach their Goal A weight and are working on a maintenance program."

The Planned Cheating lesson—the *one* lesson I am excited about.

"No self-pity," says the Genie. "You are working toward one of your current Top Four Life Goals. Do not tell me the water is rough; just bring in the ship."

As the Genie disappears, I get another text from Zach: **The roads are getting worse and worse. I am skidding everywhere. I hope this was a good idea. Be there in 10.**

Zach arrives and has salad, broccoli, fresh fruit for dessert, and his game of Wits and Wagers to play.

"Where are Richard and Beth?" he asks. I call Beth, and she picks up on the fifth ring.

"Alexis threw up, and I am not sure what is wrong with her. Anyhow, the power came back on, Jackie, so we are going to stay here."

Gulp. I need Beth and Richard here since Zach is here. "Oh, wow. I am sorry. Well, I will call you tomorrow to check on Alexis," and we hang up. Zach does not hear that conversation as he is in the kitchen, getting ready to help with the cooking.

The roads are getting worse, and Zach lives thirty minutes away. I hate to send him back out on the icy streets. I walk into the kitchen, and the weatherman on TV is saying, "Again, the roads in Nashville are dangerous. Do not, and I repeat, do not go out unless it is an emergency. Police are behind with the wrecks. I repeat, the driving conditions are extremely hazardous."

As I explain the situation with Beth to Zach, we walk to the front door to assess the situation. Both of us know the roads are not safe. "Your call," he says. "If you are too uncomfortable with me here, I will leave."

"Of course you cannot leave. The roads are terrible," I say. I am thrilled and yet uneasy at the same time at the seeming impropriety.

We cook, eat, and clean up. "Do you feel like taking a walk, or do you think it is too cold?" Zach asks. Delighted at the idea, I walk to my closet to retrieve some warm gloves, a scarf, and a heavy coat. Bundled up, we head outside.

The roads around are deserted. The snow is fresh and undisturbed, making it a gorgeous, Narnia-like wonderland. We talk about some cases from work. We talk about Mr. Hanover and his dislike of Zach breaking it off with Rachel. We talk about Zach's siblings, my siblings, and stories about when we were kids. Zach confides that someday he wants a large family, possibly six kids. The walk is maybe thirty of the best minutes of my life.

Back at the apartment, the warmth is soothing, and I put more wood on the fire. Sitting on the sofa in front of the fire, Zach and I chat some more, exchanging stories about our parents, places we would like to visit, and what we like to do in the summers. Coincidentally, both of us confess that we each want to own a lake house someday.

"Jack, I was wondering if you would like to train for a five-K run together. We could meet two nights a week after work to train and then run on Saturday mornings. I found a website that has a training schedule we could use. What do you think?" Zach asks me to train with him just like he would ask me to discuss an upcoming brief.

"I will never be able to keep up with you, Zach," I say, knowing that he has been working out for a while. The idea is very inviting, though, because not only would I get exercise off my list, I would get to hang with Zach. He will probably want to use the time talking about his new girlfriends, though.

"You will catch up quickly," he says, and we proceed to discuss the logistics of training together. I cannot think of any reason not to, so we agree to run on Monday nights, Wednesday nights, and Saturday mornings at nine.

It is getting late, and the fire is more like smoldering embers now. Glancing at Zach, I notice he is looking at me. I look away, as the eye contact makes me uncomfortable. Every neuron in my body is aflame. Every cell is ignited. However, I know I need to shake this off. I am just a friend to Zach, a legal assistant, and now a workout buddy. This is merely friendly chitchat on an icy night. Nothing more.

"I enjoyed the night, Jack," Zach says.

Again, I catch his eye. But his friendliness does not mean anything. He enjoyed a night with a good friend, a good buddy. At least I am not enough of an idiot to read anything into that sentence.

Uncomfortable though, I hop up and gather our coffee mugs, taking them to the kitchen. He follows me and I lead him to his room. We both say good night, and I head to my room.

Getting in bed, I try to sleep but have trouble because I am so excited about getting up and having breakfast with my overnight guest.

Lesson 18

Handling Food Pushers

Wednesday, December 17 Weight: 141   Pounds lost: 34   Still to go: 11

Zach got a bad cold after the ice storm, and tonight is actually the first time that we have had an opportunity to train for our run. He texts that he will be late because he had a long phone conversation with his brother in North Carolina. Then he writes: **Why don't I first go to the grocery store and buy us a couple of steaks to grill after the run?**

I write back: **Nice idea. I have ingredients for a salad/veggies. Pick up a baking potato for yourself, if you would like.** Just because I am watching carbs does not mean Zach has to.

Can I shower in your guest bath? he writes. The thought of Zach's hard body showering in my apartment makes me weak, but I hold it together.

Of course, I respond.

Putting on my running gear, I glance in the mirror. Why, I almost think it is someone else. Being down thirty-four pounds is ridiculously wonderful. I love this. I have not been this slim since I was fourteen. The exuberance I feel makes every little sacrifice of Trash Food seem pitifully small. I love my new body. I love the lightness and the confidence I feel. Why, I feel, well…sexy instead of feeling like a blimp!

Even though I am getting ready to run, I touch up my makeup a bit. After all, it *is* Zach.

"Hello, Young Jackie," the Genie says. The days of being alarmed by his sudden appearances are officially over.

"Genie, I have lost thirty-four pounds!" I scream.

"I am not surprised," he says. "What you have accomplished is normal for my *Skinny School* students. Changing how you think about food and exercise changes your body. But do not get cocky and go off the program. Furthermore, we have several important lessons to go, and I know you still want to lose those last eleven pounds."

I am still waiting for the awesome lesson on Planned Cheating.

"Tonight I want to quickly discuss Food Pushers," he says. "There are two types of Food Pushers, those who innocently suggest you eat but do not really care. And then there are the difficult kinds of people, who are trying to control you for other motives."

What minutiae he goes into.

"The first rule is to not let Food Pushers upset you," he says. "They truly have no power over whether you eat or not *except the power you give them*. So you are always in control of whether you eat or not. Never blame anyone for making you eat; only you decide whether you eat."

Somehow I feel that others have this secret control, but the Genie says they do not.

"In the case of innocent Food Pushers, they will say things like, 'This is a wedding, and it is special. Of course you are going to eat cake!' They are not trying to derail your program; they are simply uninformed."

My sisters would fall in this category.

"Just smile and say, 'The cake does look good, but I am not hungry right now. Thank you, though.' This is your mantra with Food Pushers: *'The food looks good, but I am not hungry right now—or, I would rather eat X. Thank you, though.'* If they push you ten times, say that ten times. Do not get mad because honestly, they do not understand. Most Food Pushers are the innocent type."

Beth is like this, too.

"And then," he says, "there are the serious Food Pushers, who want to control you. These folks take a more solid backbone to stand up to. But again, say and repeat the mantra: 'The food looks good, but I am not hungry right now—or, I would rather eat X. Thank you, though.'"

I guess I could say that.

"I have prepared some Quart Bags for you along with a salad and a recipe of Genie Lasagna," he says and disappears.

There is a knock at the door, and when I open it, there is Zach in his sweat pants, a hat, and gloves. We quickly season the steaks, scrub his potato and put it in the oven, and then head out the door for our interval training. Gasping for air, I have to slow down more than I had hoped. However, Zach does not seem annoyed at all at my out-of-shape lungs. In fact, he insists that I will gain endurance soon.

After our workout, Zach showers in the guest bath while I shower in my bathroom. He comes out of the shower wearing jeans and a T-shirt, towel-drying his wet hair. The scent of the soap on his skin jolts me, but again, I manage to hide it. It is a little overwhelming, Zach Boltz, showering in my apartment, getting ready to cook together alone.

Quickly, I apply a little makeup. At least I have good skin. I throw on some jeans and an old University of Memphis sweatshirt. In the past, I felt the need to wear long shirts to cover my bootie, but with this weight loss, I feel comfortable with a normal top. It feels great to not be concerned with hiding my body. Hiding my weight under tent-like shirts has been upsetting for thirteen years. The time and angst I have spent trying to hide my weight are ridiculous. I cannot believe this might really be over.

Moving into the kitchen, Zach and I begin to chop and laugh and chat. The steaks are absolutely delicious (I only eat half of mine, saving half for tomorrow's lunch), and Zach does not seem in a hurry to go. His phone rings and it is his brother, but Zach says he will call him back.

"Why don't you take it?" I say. "I will start on the dishes."

"No, he only wants to talk about my trip to visit him again, and I am a little uncomfortable about it all."

"Why are you uncomfortable? Your brother, Jonathan, is one of your favorite people," I say. I found this out the night we walked in the snow. We both stand up and begin carrying dishes into the kitchen.

"Yes, that is true," Zach says. "Jonathan and his wife, Shelley, asked me to come to North Carolina to visit them on New Year's Eve, and I agreed. Now they are trying to...well, Shelley is trying to...set me up on a date with one of her friends. I guess this friend has been out of the country and is coming back in town for New Year's Eve."

"Back in the country? Where has she been?" I ask, feeling a little kick in my stomach, thinking about Zach going on a date.

"She has been helping out in an orphanage in Romania," Zach says. Now this is the kind of girl that Zach needs, not the country club socialite that Rachel was.

"Wow, she sounds like a nice person," I say, struggling to sound normal. I know it will just be a matter of time until a lovely girl like this captures his heart. "What else did your brother tell you about her?" I ask, not prying but simply making friendly conversation. Zach rinses off the dishes while I load them in the dishwasher.

"Well, eh...Jonathan said she has been a best friend of Shelley's since grade school."

Dang. Zach already told me that Shelley went to one of those la-di-da uppity private schools, like Rachel. This girl is also a blue blood like Zach.

"Did he say anything else about her?" I ask. I guess I might be prying now. Putting dishwashing detergent in the dispenser, I try to act only mildly interested.

"Well, he said, uh, that she was, uh...a runner-up in the Miss North Carolina contest," he says.

If learning that this girl worked at an orphanage punched me before, this statement sends me into lockdown shock. A girl with a great heart, blue blood, *and* a beauty-queen background? Oh, my. He needs to start shopping now for the engagement ring.

"Wow," is all I can think to say. Who can compete with a girl who works with orphans and is a beauty queen? I cannot remember feeling so unworthy in a long time. Of course, Zach's sister-in-law wants to fix him up. I can already tell they will be soul mates.

The contrast between a Miss North Carolina beauty queen and me is the distance between the earth and the sun. My averageness screams. Jackie Average—that should be my middle name. Zach-types don't marry their hard-working, average legal assistants. They run and train for 5Ks with them. They marry runners-up in beauty contests.

"We run again on Saturday morning, okay?" Zach asks, as we finish wiping off the counters. I say okay, and he leaves. I watch him walk to his car through the peephole. His strong body, his strong mind, his well-bred family...all out of my league. Sure, good ole Jackie, good for training, counseling, and being an awesome legal assistant. But now he is going to fall in love with Miss North Carolina Runner-Up, with all her teased hair, dark eyeliner, and soft heart for orphans. A grief fills my stomach and heart. The grief is not as intense as when I lost my mom in the car wreck, but nevertheless, it is a severe grief. I know it is just a matter of time until Zach falls in love with a perfect girl like that.

Lesson 19

The Champion Mind-set, Revisited

Tuesday, December 24   Weight: 139   Pounds lost: 36   Still to lose: 9

Zach and I ran twice again after that first run, the next Saturday and the next Monday night. We talked about music, how we each felt about education (public, private, or homeschooling), about which novels we have read and liked (he likes Michael Connelly, too), and about a zillion other topics. If I am supposed to be on a self-imposed program to get over Zach, it is not working. And now he is going to North Carolina for New Year's, and then the fairy-tale romance will begin.

Zach and I did not run last week as I caught Zach's cold. I had hoped we could have somehow hung out, but we did not. Zach did text me a lot while I was sick, though, to see how I was feeling. Now our runs will have to be put off again as today is Christmas Eve, and I leave for Memphis later today.

The office is closing shop at noon as we are having a big Christmas party. Eva was in charge of planning the menu. We drew names at the office, and I got Eva's name. I got her some Katy Perry perfume called Purr that smells divine. Richard drew my name, and obviously Beth bought the present. It was a knife from Williams-Sonoma. Beth knows what a little cook I have become.

"Jackie, try one of these brownies," Eva says. "They are absolutely the best."

They do look good, but brownies are not on my Daily Plan.

"No, thank you," I say.

"You cannot always be on a diet!" she says in front of everyone. "It is Christmas. Isn't that a little obsessive to never cheat? Even on Christmas?"

My blood pressure is rising. Talking about my diet and my eating in front of everyone is embarrassing. What did the Genie tell me to say?

"Well, I don't know, but…"

Getting a brownie off the tray, she offers it to me and says, "Here, just take a bite and see how it tastes."

The pressure of the group watching me makes me feel sick. "Well, I know it looks good, and I do appreciate you doing all the planning for lunch, Eva, but I would rather eat the turkey and raw veggies. Thank you, though." My heart rate must be two hundred, but actually, that response works. Eva relents and is backing off.

Filling my plate with turkey, ham, raw veggies, some dip, and a few nuts, I tell myself that life is not in Christmas Trash Food. Parties and food pushers like Eva are difficult but not unsurmountable.

As I gather my belongings to leave, Zach says there is a Christmas bonus in my check. I smile and thank him. I sort of expected that, to be honest. "Are you going straight home?" he asks. I guess he is just asking because the weather forecast calls for ice.

"Yes," I say, "but I am leaving shortly to drive to Memphis." I leave the office and feel down. No *ho, ho, ho* for me, but rather *bah humbug*. Another Christmas, alone again. Eva chatted up Zach nonstop at the Christmas party, but he only responded in a polite manner. Eva is not Zach's type by any standard, but I am pretty sure Ms. North Carolina Runner-Up is a perfect match.

After arriving home, I finish packing. It is time to make the three-hour drive to Memphis, so I can arrive early enough to go to the Christmas Eve service at Jessica's church. However, I still need to wrap the eight presents I am taking to my sisters' kids.

As I look at my suitcase, a heavy discouragement descends upon me. I have lost a lot of weight, yes, but that does not guarantee smooth sailing through life. Disappointments still hurt. There is no denying that I feel down…and sad. I am single, it is Christmas, and my boss is getting ready to fall madly in love with Ms. Runner-Up. I will never find a soul mate. The idea that an ice cream cone would make me feel better comes to mind.

Listening to myself whine, I realize I am having a true pity party. Pathetic! Time to quit that! Intentionally taking my mind off my problems, I begin to think about what else I need to pack to take to Memphis.

Walking into my closet to get the supplies needed to wrap the presents, I find all eight of my presents already wrapped. **The Genie is standing there with a Santa cap on.**

"Hello, Young Jackie, and Merry Christmas," the Genie says. He looks rather ridiculous, but his high energy is a nice contrast to how depleted I feel.

"Today we will revisit a topic that we have previously discussed many times, but because this topic is of paramount importance, I want to take a full lesson to discuss it," he says.

Hmm. I wonder what topic it could be. Packing? Tracking?

"Our topic is the Mind-set of a Champion," he says.

He's right; I thought we had covered that.

"Life is rarely a yellow brick road," the Genie begins. "It is more often pot-holes, detours, and traffic jams. Events happen you do not like, people break promises, people disappoint you, and unpleasant surprises are guaranteed."

Yeah, what a bummer all that is.

"In the scheme of life, you can count on adversity, turmoil, bedlam, distress, pandemonium, strife, agitations, and mix-ups," he says. "Life is unpredictable, and disorder and disturbance will appear. Your plan will not work out. This is not surprising; this is merely what every human experiences sometime in life."

Really? My expectations and mental picture of life is a summer holiday with flowery meadows and sunshine. This might begin to explain why I am repeatedly disappointed.

"When normal life situations such as these happen, most people make excuses, complain about delays, postpone doing what they know they need to do, become tired, blocked, stressed, busy, or overwhelmed."

Ha-ha, yes—that is exactly how I respond.

"Turbulence, tragedy, setbacks, failure, and darkness are a part of life, Young Jackie. It is guaranteed that life will cut you open. As you know, in life you do not get everything you want, so why be unhappy and overreact when this *normal, set-in-cement* aspect of life shows up?" he asks.

Eh, I didn't know there was another way to react to unwanted circumstances.

"Quit expecting life to treat you as if you are a princess. Much of your inner turmoil is because your expectations are that life is a river float trip down a smooth, slow river in an inner tube with a cooler attached."

That does sound kind of fun—as long as I am skinny while floating in that inner tube. Inner tubes mean bathing suits.

"When your world falls apart, have an inner resolve that you will lean in and take *action to solve your dilemmas* instead of starting the debate about whether you are going to go off your *Skinny School* program and self-medicate. Your resolve must be to stay on the *Skinny School* program—regardless! When the unwanted appears and the temptation to self-medicate arises, double up on the basics: *read your Ruby Journal, ditch sweets and starches, track, plan, shop, prep, prepare your Quart Bags and soup, wait until you are hungry to eat, stop at a five, analyze your failure, and plan your exercise.*"

The basics, yes, the beautiful basics. How quickly I forget.

"Champions mentally prepare for the difficulties ahead," he says. "They develop a will of iron that no matter what—no matter what—no matter what, they will persist. They throw excuses like 'just this once' and 'this time is special' into the deep abyss. Champions cheerfully face unwanted circumstances with iron spines and with action. They know that the only way to do something spectacular is to use colossal effort. They do not expect an easy road. Their secrets are work, action, and plans. They succeed by analyzing failure, regrouping, and continuing. Even though they often do not feel ready, Champions begin. They realize that all of life is not supposed to feel comfortable, and *on the other side of persistence is glory and victory.* Champions do not complain that they do not have what they want; they take mammoth action to go after it. They know persistence and action are the genius and the power. So like these Champions, Young Jackie, conquer the *Skinny School* program by instructing your mind to repeatedly perform the basics. And not tomorrow, but today. Now. This second."

In the past, I have had a million excuses why I needed to eat for comfort or entertainment, but the Genie wants me to draw a line in the sand and say, "No more."

"React to turbulence with calm logic, humility, and honesty, and do not go off your program. Begin to have tolerance for unknown obstacles that will arise. When you are tempted to medicate your emotions to soothe yourself, respond to your Demanding Child with outrageous indignation."

I feel like I have joined the Marines.

"Genie, all this talk of overcoming and standing up to resistance still seems hard to me," I say.

"Hard? Hard? Are you kidding me?" he says. "This is one of the most important secrets in life that humans fail to grasp. Just like you have to go through conflict to get to intimacy in relationships, you have to go through self-discipline and self-mastery to get to exhilaration in accomplishment. Humans want all the *delight of life* without paying the price. It is absolutely absurd. Push yourself through hard workouts. Do not eat sweets or starches. Do the work to plan and prep, and on the other side is waking up and seeing a small, fit body in the mirror. This is the way to live: *putting oneself through the pain of self-mastery and self-discipline* as this *leads to exhilaration*. Pain first, then the prize. Pain *must precede* the prize. This is the only intelligent way to live. Press through hard times, do not cave, and exhilaration will follow. Self-mastery and self-discipline are your best friends, taking you to emotional well-being. Honestly, it shocks me that anyone would choose to live any differently."

For months, Genie has talked about the "flip" or the "click" when I get it. I think it just happened. I mean, I have been wailing and fussing about how hard this *Skinny School* program is, how deprived I have felt, and instead, I now see that self-mastery and self-discipline are the on-the-floor, front-row tickets. They are the coveted traits! They are the secrets, the splendor, the triumph. How my heart has hated discipline, but that was because I did not understand that it is the mysterious and obscure tunnel to the grandeur of thinness! These thoughts are definitely going in my Ruby Journal. Why, of course this makes sense. Self-mastery and self-discipline are difficult in the moment, but I have to pass through that swamp to get to the promised land of one of my current Top Four Life Goals, magnificent skinniness.

"This is how Champions train themselves to think," he says, "and this is how I expect you to control your thoughts. You are the emperor of a vast empire, your mind. Take charge of your thoughts. Behead the troublemakers. You do this by reading the meaningful sentences in your Ruby Journal and rereading them until they belong to you. *Thinking the right thoughts is the true secret to being thin.* I left a couple Genie Steak Rollups in your fridge to take as a snack on your drive to Memphis. Merry Christmas, Young Jackie," he says and disappears.

Any discouragement I possessed earlier has completely vanished, and I feel pumped and empowered to handle any oncoming discord or turbulence. My resolve is strong. I do not feel vulnerable to my sappy, whiney lower nature. Maybe I can also apply some of this amazing thinking to my discouragement when Zach falls in love with Ms. Runner-Up.

And so much for that ice cream cone that I was considering.

There is a knock at the door. Who could that be? I peep through the peephole, and it is Zach! What is he doing here?

"Zach!" I say, in a surprised tone. "I wasn't expecting you." He has a beautifully wrapped present in his hands.

"I have something more for you," he says. His olive skin has a warm, robust look that is in stark contrast to the blizzardy feel of the outdoors. His dark hair is a little overgrown and therefore more wavy than usual. His ability to ignite my chemistry has activated, and I try to contain it. I feel faint just looking at him.

"You got me something?" I ask, happy and delighted but trying to hide it.

"Yes, I did," and that small grin of his creeps across his face.

Almost feeling intoxicated, I do not know what to say. I just stand there.

"Open it," he urges.

"Okay," I say as he walks inside my apartment. He is still dressed from work, and his Brooks Brothers charcoal pants and Johnston Murphy shoes fit his no-nonsense personality. I am already in jeans and tennis shoes, ready to make the drive to Elvis's and my hometown.

We both sit down on the sofa, and I start unwrapping the present.

What? What? Oh. My. Goodness! It's a Canon EOS 70 D Digital SLR camera. This is the thousand-dollar camera I was oohing over that Bodybuilder Chad had when the office went ice skating the day of my wreck.

"This is waaaay too nice of a present," I blurt out.

"Great assistants need great presents," he says.

"But you already gave me a generous bonus in my check," I say, shell-shocked.

"I thought you would like it," he says, acting like a five-year-old boy who just gave his teacher a present.

Zach could have bought this camera for his business and then let me use his to take photos. He did not have to give me such a fabulous present. This is really nice...incredibly nice.

"I do not know what to say, except, well...except thank you, and...I absolutely love it." I am not sure how I have the nerve to do this, but I reach over and hug him. And he hugs me back. In fact, he hugs hard and long and does not let me go for at least five seconds, maybe six.

I wait until he loosens his grip, and then I pull back.

"I am glad you like it," Zach says, neither one of us looking at each other, both obviously embarrassed from that long, lingering hug.

"I did not get you anything," I say. I wanted to—believe me, I wanted to. But since we drew names at the office, it seemed wrong to buy him something.

"That is why I did not give it to you until now," he says. "I did not want you to give me anything. You working for me is the best gift I got this year."

I look away first. My face must be as red as Santa's suit. The gift is just because I am an awesome assistant, I remind myself. Nothing more.

Fiddling with the camera gives me an excuse to not look at Zach. I am not sure what to make of this moment. Again, I wrestle my thoughts down. He is just grateful for me to work for him, I tell myself.

As I walk Zach to the door, he turns around before he exits. We look at each other again. "Merry Christmas, Jack," he says, still not moving.

"Merry Christmas, Zach," I say.

Again, he does not move. I think I may pass out. What is he doing, taking so long? Why is he just standing there, gazing at me?

Finally, he turns to leave. He walks to his car, gets in, and drives away.

What was that? What was that lingering and that staring? I felt like the chemistry between us took up the whole room. No, more like the chemistry between us took up the whole planet.

My discouragement has lifted, and now it is replaced with royal confusion.

Lesson 20

The Secret of Soup

Friday, December 27   Weight: 139   Pounds Lost: 36   Still to lose: 9

Christmas in Memphis was uneventful. All my little nieces and nephews made the holiday fun but exhausting. I was glad to be there but also glad to come back to my life in Nashville. Zach texted me several times while I was in Memphis, but they were light-hearted jokes or casual observances about things we are both interested in. He did not mention the hug when he would not let me go, nor did he mention the chemistry that took over the whole planet when he was standing in the doorway, saying good-bye. Thinking about things in hindsight, I realize I was the only one feeling the chemistry, and he was merely being a good friend. I am such a wishful loser. But still, I cannot quit thinking about Zach leaving next Tuesday to go fall in love with Miss Runner-Up.

Eva walks up to my desk in her short black skirt, textured hose, tight leopard-print sweater, and earrings that hang down four inches. "How was Memphis, Jackie? Did your sisters set you up with anyone while you were there?"

Knowing that Zach can hear every word, I cringe.

"No, they didn't," I respond, looking down at my keyboard and hoping she will go away.

"Don't they know any cute guys? Now that you have lost so much weight, I thought they would set you up on a blind date," she says.

Again realizing that Zach is listening to every word, I feel sick. I would like to shoo her away, like one does a fly. Ignoring her, she persists. "Has your weight loss affected your dating life?"

Enough. Totally enough. Getting up from my desk, I say, "I don't know, Eva, but I have got some work to do, so we will have to talk later," and I take an armful of files to the copy machine room, like I am going to make copies. Fortunately, she does not follow me. I walk into the copy machine room and want to kick the wall. Why does she feel like she can ask such intrusive questions? I hate that I have to work with her. And I hate that I am single, and I hate that Zach is getting ready to meet a true gem of a girl. I hate-hate-hate it all. The thought of Trash Food comes to mind. I feel ridiculously upset and discouraged.

So that I can have a little privacy, I shut the door. **But not surprisingly, the Genie appears and offers me some hot vegetable-beef soup.** Inhaling the soup, I notice my severe anxiety subsides somewhat. Learning to dial down emotions without food is *not* an acquired skill yet, but at least I am dialing down mammoth emotions without Trash Food.

"As you know, no one can hear or see me except you," he begins. "Today we will talk about the Secret of Soup. Last lesson, I admonished you in a military fashion to acquire the mind-set of a Champion. The lesson today is softer, as it is about comfort."

My kind of lesson, comfort! And I just experienced what he is talking about when I ate the vegetable-beef soup and quickly felt better.

"Soup has been a favorite among humans for centuries," he begins. "Nutritious and filling, soup calms nerves and soothes ruffled feathers. Soup is satisfying and can be a huge help in your *Skinny School* program. Collect recipes for soups that are allowed on your eating regime, ones without pasta, potatoes, or other starchy foods. Soups are another tool that can help you stay on your *Skinny School* program."

When Eva pulls her stuff, I need all the tricks I can get to calm down.

"Of course, my first preference is for you to wait until you are hungry to eat," he says, "but there will be times, like right now, when you will need some comfort, and a cup of soup is often just the right item to help you."

As much as he barks about waiting until I am hungry to eat, I am glad he realizes I am human and that sometimes it is absolutely necessary to dial down feelings with food. And soup, I now realize, is a great choice.

"There is a recipe of Genie Weight Loss Vegetable Soup in your fridge at home," he says and disappears.

Wow, what a short lesson. But even in that small amount of time, I feel much more composed. I return to my office, and Eva enters again. She announces that "the new lawyer that Daddy hired starts today" and that "he will be here soon." She adds one more comment: "He is drop-dead gorgeous." We all knew that the Simpson Law Firm has been steadily growing over the last year and that Attorney Simpson has been on the lookout for another hotshot young personal-injury attorney. Eva says the new lawyer, Thomas Fleetwood, is bringing his legal assistant, Amanda, with him, who is also supposed to help Attorney Simpson, since, ahem, his daughter cannot seem to understand common legal words like *liability* and *uninsured motorist*.

Thirty minutes later, Eva walks into my office again, and behind her is a thirty-year-old, six-foot-two, auburn-haired Greek god. He has on a beautiful gray flannel suit, a white starched shirt, and a gorgeous paisley teal tie.

"This is Thomas Fleetwood," Eva says. "And this is Jackie Holbrook." Eva is falling all over herself, smiling, touching herself, sashaying around.

The Greek god smiles. Nice teeth. "I hear you are the superstar legal assistant who can write briefs," he says. Do I detect dimples?

I modestly smile but am pleased my reputation has preceded me. However, now that I have lost thirty-six pounds, men treat me differently. Handsome men notice me in a way they never have in twenty-eight years.

"Nice to meet you, Thomas," I say, not being able to think of anything clever. These Ryan Reynolds–look-alike men do that to me.

"My legal assistant from my old firm, Amanda, is going to work here too, but she won't be here until later today," he says. "Maybe you can teach her some of your tricks." And again, he flashes the dimples. Thomas keeps smiling and lingering. This feels nice. *I am* so *not used to this.*

Zach walks out of his office and shakes hands with Thomas, and it is immediately obvious they already know each other. "Jackie is not only a great brief writer," Zach says, "but if you need some help understanding a law, she is your go-to person here." They are both playing with me now, but I like people noticing my brains. They are all I have had worth noticing for many years.

Eva apparently does not like the attention to not be centered on her, so she begins to make some irrelevant comments about the coffee, bouncing around like a puppy wanting to be petted.

Thomas glances at me one more time. One more flash of the dimples. I can already tell he sort of likes me. I am glad to have some new blood in this office. Zach is getting ready to fall in love with Miss Runner-Up, and I am going to need a new friend. A new handsome, thirty-year-old male friend.

Lunchtime rolls around, and Thomas strolls up to my desk. "What does everyone here do for lunch?" he asks, his eyes twinkling. Simultaneously Zach walks out of his office and lays some papers to be filed on my desk. Upon hearing Thomas's question, he quickly retreats to his office.

I cannot exactly describe what it is, but the dance of the eyes, the flash of the dimples, and the tone of Thomas's voice all mix together, and I can read that Thomas is interested in me. Take that, Zachy boy. I may be an awesome assistant, but possibly now, I am also able to attract handsome men.

Smiling up at Thomas, I say, "I bring my lunch most days, but when I don't, I go to Panera Bread around the corner."

"Did you bring your lunch today?" he asks, as I again notice the twinkle in his eye. I like this. I really do.

"Yes, but I am tired of turkey. I could go for one of Panera Bread's salads," I say, hoping that Zach is listening.

"Great," Thomas says. "Name the time."

"What about if we leave in fifteen minutes?" I ask.

Thomas returns to his office, and right before I gather my purse to leave, Zach comes back out of his office. He looks intently at me and does not say a word for a few seconds. I smile sweetly at him.

"Are you sore from your exercise?" he asks, obviously just making conversation.

"No," I say, as I get my purse and start to stand up. "I feel great, absolutely great." And with that, I walk out of the office and down the hall to meet Thomas.

At lunch, Thomas is very funny and has many hilarious stories to tell. What a stroke of good luck to have Thomas now working at the office. It will help me keep my mind off Zach since he is only a couple days away from falling in love with Ms. Runner-Up.

Returning to the office after lunch, Thomas and I both get busy working. Thomas's legal assistant from his old law firm, Amanda, arrives after lunch to meet everyone. I already like her cheerful disposition, and to add to that, she is friends with Beth and Richard.

"My husband and I both love the Willifords," she says. "We should all hang out some time. Are you dating anyone?"

At this moment, Thomas walks in and watches my face to see what I am going to answer. "No, not at the moment," I say.

"Well, we will have to fix you up, so the six of us can go to dinner!" Amanda suggests.

"And if you cannot think of anyone else," Thomas jumps in, "you can substitute me." Amanda looks at Thomas quizzically, and then it dawns on her: he is interested in me!

Zach walks out of his office and is bumbling through the files for some reason. I am not sure what he is doing.

"What about New Year's Eve?" Amanda suggests. "Are you two busy? I could call Beth and Richard and see if they are." Thomas raises his eyebrows at me as if to ask, "Okay with you?"

I sweetly smile back and say, "I am game."

Now this is a scream. Zach is watching a very attractive guy be interested in me. Maybe I am not just a fat ole legal assistant anymore who is only good for writing briefs. Maybe I am worth taking out on New Year's Eve! Yeah, Zach Boltz! Pay attention. Other men now think I am attractive!

Again, Zach is shuffling the files, something he never does.

"Let me text Beth, and I will get back to you," Amanda says. She does, and it is all set up for New Year's Eve. The six of us are going out together!

It is now past five, and I get my coat, ready to leave for the weekend. Zach flies out to North Carolina tomorrow morning to visit his brother. I stick my head in his doorway and say a sweet, "See you next year!"

He does not smile, but says, "Yeah, Jack, see you next year."

Happily, I turn and walk out. Go ahead and fall in love with Ms. Runner-Up, Zach. Maybe I will fall in love, too.

Lesson 21

How Alcohol Affects Your Metabolism

Tuesday, December 31   Weight: 138   Pounds lost: 37   Still to lose: 8

Zach texted me a couple times over the weekend, but they were all about inane things, such as his brother's kids and the weather.

It is now New Year's Eve, and I am waiting on Thomas to arrive to pick me up. Thomas is ridiculously good looking, but I have noticed that he is quite the talker and is not that great of a listener. Maybe he will do better as he gets to know me.

Looking into the mirror, I realize I have never looked so good in my life. These black, shiny pants are ridiculously slenderizing, and I love this shiny, black top with all the rhinestones. My confidence is up like never before. I love being a semi-thin woman! This feeling is something I have missed out on for thirteen years, just because I did not know the path out of the Food Dungeon. Oh, what I would give to have known these *Skinny School* secrets thirteen years ago!

Arriving at the New Year's Eve party, I am in high spirits with my new cute date. Thomas and I dance and dance. Thomas is very likeable, but he does monopolize the conversation. I cannot worry about that right now. Maybe most great-looking guys do that.

From inside my purse, I see a light flash from my phone. That is strange. **Who could be calling me on New Year's Eve? Oh, heavens, it is the Genie.** I go to the bathroom to take the call.

"Tonight I want to talk to you about alcohol and its effect on weight loss," the Genie begins.

"But Genie, I do not drink," I say, noticing, however, that almost everyone else at this party is drinking alcohol. But really, is this not absolutely the most ridiculous time ever for a lesson, during a party? And on the phone!

"You still need this information," he says, "as someday I hope you will help others with their weight." I know he wants me to help others, but I have not felt comfortable doing that until, well, maybe soon.

"Alcohol is processed differently from food in the liver," he begins. "When the liver recognizes alcohol, it immediately focuses on breaking down the acetate in the alcohol. What this tends to do is to *dramatically reduce one's metabolism*. An occasional glass of wine is usually not a problem, but if someone drinks very much, it is quite a hindrance to one's weight loss."

I think of one of my sisters, Chloe, and her incessant exercise, as well as her careful attention to not eating sweets and starches. Immediately I understand why she is not losing weight.

"Some women love a glass of wine even more than a piece of chocolate cake," the Genie says. "The relaxing and comforting glass of wine is a ritual in many women's lives, and giving that up for weight loss is a tough decision."

At 5:00 p.m. every day, Chloe pops that cork and pours her wine. I have even wondered if she has a drinking problem, since she seems to make sure that wine is always available.

"Many women would rather be five or eight pounds overweight instead of giving up their daily alcohol," he says. "It is a decision, though, of what one wants more: thinness or the daily relaxation. It seems almost impossible for women to be as slim as they want without severely limiting their alcohol."

At least I do not have to fight drinking alcohol. Fighting to *not eat* for comfort and stimulation is hard enough.

"What is helpful to some women who truly want to be thin is to learn to replace the five p.m. ritual with having another yummy drink," he says. "Red raspberry herbal tea with stevia or honey caramel herbal tea with stevia and a little whipping cream are delicious alternatives. Granted, they do not relax one like alcohol does, but they do offer calming benefits. A woman who really loves and depends on her wine, though, will have a hard time giving it up. Only when she wants thinness *more* will she be willing to give up a pleasure that she so greatly enjoys. Since both thinness and having a daily cocktail are usually of high importance in many women's lives, they will have to be very intentional about handling this conflict. It is a difficult decision to give up a pleasure that is rated a nine—like wine—to go after a pleasure rated ten—like thinness."

I get giving up pleasure. I have given up the pleasure that is rated nine to me—desserts—because I am going after a higher pleasure, thinness. Honestly though, wanting both haunts me all the time. I have to remember that this sacrifice is temporary, and when I get to my goal weight, I can add back a couple desserts a week. Remembering that all Champions give up *good* things to get the *best* things is helpful.

"I hear women whine that they want to be thin more than anything," he says, "but when it comes time to give up wine, they resist."

Thinking about Chloe, I think she would rather be eight pounds over her goal weight than give up wine.

"We will discuss Planned Cheating soon," the Genie says, "but know that after women reach their goal weight, they can have cheat items two or three times a week. Not two or three cheat *meals*, but two to three cheat *items*. The cheat items I am talking about are bread, alcohol, or dessert. Eventually, a woman can have a couple glasses of wine a week and still stay thin. Again, it is a choice a woman must figure out. If a woman doesn't want to give up her daily glass of wine, then she either must be content with being a few pounds over her Goal A weight, with severely restricting her food, or with doing an intense amount of exercise."

Ah ha, I love it when he talks about adding back bread and dessert! Yippee!

"There are a couple Genie Bacon Cheeseburgers in your fridge. Happy New Year," the Genie says and hangs up.

Returning to the crowd, I see Thomas, and he motions for me to come over to him. Just as I reach him, my phone lights up again. What does the Genie want now? Oh, my—it is Zach!

"Excuse me a second, Thomas," I say, turning my back and answering the call.

"Hello?"

"Yeah, well...hey, Jack. I just...uh...wanted to say...uh...Happy New Year."

I am not sure what is up.

Walking a few steps away from Thomas, I ask, "Where is Miss Runner-Up?"

He laughs at *Miss Runner-Up.* "She is inside with my brother and his wife. I just stepped outside to call you."

He stepped outside to call me right before midnight on New Year's Eve? The music is getting louder. The guy on the microphone says it is two minutes until the New Year arrives, so everyone should fill their glasses to toast.

"How is your night with Thomas?" he asks. This seems like a rather odd question.

"Fine," I say. "How is your night with Miss Runner-Up?"

"Well, she is okay," he says. "She just told me she is moving to Nashville in January to take a job as the children's director at the First Presbyterian Church. Actually, she is coming next weekend to look for an apartment. It was a surprise."

Uh, she is what? Miss Runner-Up is moving to Nashville? Why, this was not expected. She got that job, and now she has already found the prince of Nashville to date? Zach is probably calling me so that I will invite her to stay with me next weekend while she apartment shops. Why, that is why he is calling me! He wants me to invite his new girlfriend to stay with me. Well, he can jump off a cliff. I am not inviting any beauty queen to stay with me. Pathetic, Zach. I draw the line here.

Thomas looks at me and motions for me to fill my glass as it is almost time to toast. "Jack," Thomas almost yells, "It is fifteen seconds until New Year's. Tell them you will call them back."

"When did Thomas start calling you *Jack*?" Zach asks.

I don't answer because Thomas is walking toward me and would hear me.

"Ten...nine...eight..." counts down the guy on the microphone.

"I just wanted you to know that…" Zach's voice trails off.

"Know what?" I ask with an edge to my voice. You want me to know that you are falling in love with Miss Runner-Up? Is that what this is all about, Zach? You want me to ask her to stay with me? Good ole Jackie. Fat or thin, she is good for whatever you need.

"Four…three…two…" yells the guy on the microphone.

It is midnight. Thomas reaches for me and, unaware that I am still on the phone, loudly says, "It is time for a New Year's kiss…"

"We will talk later, Jack," Zach says and hangs up. He heard Thomas say that. Good. I am glad he heard it because I am sick of his nice long stares. Sure, good ole Jackie, she will work to the bone for you, won't she, Zach? But not anymore. I have had enough. I am not your servant, helping you with your girlfriends. And I am tired of being used. Thomas likes me. I am going to see if I can forget about you, Zach, and fall for Thomas.

The confetti is everywhere and everyone is kissing. Thomas smiles at me and says, "Okay, I get it. I will just kiss you on the cheek." He does and then says, "Who were you talking to?"

"Should old acquaintance be forgot…" is booming on the speakers.

"Just a friend," I reply.

He smiles and lets it go. "I expect to have some competition with a girl like you, Jack, and I want you to know I am up for it." Again, he flashes those dimples. Thomas is very sweet, and definitely I could date him. He is smart and nice, and he really likes me. Maybe I can get used to him talking so much. Anyhow, I am sick of Zach putting knives in my heart.

"Let's dance," Thomas says, as he grabs my hand and leads me to the dance floor. Actually, dancing as a semiskinny girl is quite a lot of fun. I have missed out on many enjoyable activities over the last thirteen years because I was carrying around all that extra weight.

The thought of Zach stings, but Adam Levine's "Bang Bang" makes me temporarily forget my boss as I give in to the festivity of the music, the night, and the attractive, auburn-haired man with dimples. I let Thomas know I like him. And at the door, I actually do let him kiss me. Not too many fireworks for me, but hey, this may take a little time. At least he is not using me! Zach can just marry his orphan-loving, tiara-wearing new girlfriend, but he will not be using me anymore.

Lesson 22

Planned Cheating

Friday, January 23   *Weight: 136*   *Pounds lost: 39*   *Still to lose: 6*

After Zach arrived home from North Carolina, I told him that I was not going to be able to run with him anymore. When he asked why, I explained that Thomas invited me to play league tennis on Monday nights as well as go to a class on apologetics at his church on Wednesday nights. Zach stared at me for a full five seconds and then said, "Sure, I understand," and quickly walked back to his office. We have not said one word about anything that was not business related since he returned from North Carolina, over three weeks ago. He and Ms. Runner-Up must almost be engaged by now.

"Jack, the Dobbins brief is coming up. We need to work on it," Zach says.

"I can this morning," I say.

"I can't," he says. "I have a Benefit Review Conference."

"Well, what about this afternoon?" I offer.

"I can't then, either," he says. "I hate to impose on your Saturday, but could we meet tomorrow morning for breakfast and work on it then? I hate to put it off until Monday."

Thomas and I are going out at 2:00 p.m., but I am free in the morning. I am not sure why he did not bring this up earlier in the week, but maybe he was too busy.

"Sure, I will meet you for breakfast," I say. I mean, this *is* my job.

"I will pick you up at nine a.m., and then we will decide where we want to eat," he says.

Saturday morning comes, and Zach knocks on the door, unlike most guys, who would text, **Here.**

We drive to the Noshville restaurant, order breakfast, and work on the brief for fifteen minutes—and then he says we are through. The waitress pours us a second cup of coffee.

"What are you doing today?" he asks. I am a little surprised at the invasive question, but I let it go.

"Thomas and I are playing tennis at two, and then we are going to dinner after that," I say.

"Great," he says, "then you have time to go look at the house that I am thinking about buying," he says.

Oh, dang. This is so normal. Zach wants the brain of Jackie to look at the house that he is going to buy where he and Ms. Runner-Up will have their children. Wonderful.

"I don't know, Zach. I need to—"

He interrupts. "You just said you do not have to be ready for tennis until two. It is only ten a.m. I want to get your opinion."

I know, I know. Zach loves my brain and opinions. I am Jackie, the smart girl who can write briefs and give good opinions. I cannot think of an excuse, so we get in his car and start the drive.

I am kind of sick about Zach getting a house because it is obvious to me that he is thinking about settling down, since he is with Ms. Runner-Up. I have tried to get over Zach, but moments like this tell me I have not yet succeeded.

We drive to Franklin, a suburb of Nashville. The house is beyond wonderful. One story, trees in the yard, a fenced back yard, and a porch with a swing. The cuteness of the house makes me sadder.

Thomas is such a nice guy, and six months ago, I would not have believed that I could date someone of Thomas's caliber. But thinking about Zach buying a house makes me deeply sad. And Thomas talks *waaay* too much.

Zach knows the lockbox key code, and we walk in.

The house being a little older house, I expect the inside to be tired. But someone has already updated this little dollhouse. Obviously some walls have been knocked down, and the house is airy and open. The kitchen has been completely renovated as have the two bathrooms. It is only eighteen hundred square feet, but it is a great house. Peeking into the backyard, I notice it is filled with dogwoods and azaleas. There are rosebushes and hedges for privacy. What a romantic hideaway.

"What do you think?" he asks.

"I love it," I honestly say. "I absolutely love it." Even though I am trying to be cheerful, I realize something very sad is going on in my heart. Even I am surprised at the grief I feel.

"You do?" he asks with enthusiasm.

"Yes, I really love it." Again, I feel punched in the stomach, thinking of Zach getting up in his silk pajamas with Ms. Runner-Up fixing him coffee and eggs.

"They are asking too much for it," Zach says, "but I am going to counter offer."

"You? Negotiate? Surely not!" I tease him, with both of us knowing that he is one of the best legal negotiators in town.

Zach's cell rings, and it is the weekend answering service with a potential new personal-injury case. Zach excuses himself and goes out on the front porch where the reception is better to take the call.

Opening a closet door to further check out the house, I am startled, as there is the Genie.

"No worries," he says. "As you know, no one can hear or see me except you."

Feeling down about Zach's new love nest with his future wife, I am glad to have the Genie get my mind on something else.

"Today we will discuss Planned Cheating and Maintenance. It is always a favorite topic of my clients." I have been looking forward to this topic for weeks. I think of how much I would have liked a biscuit this morning at the Noshville restaurant.

"There are two topics to discuss concerning Planned Cheating," he says. "One is Planned Cheating while you are still trying to get to your goal. And topic two is Planned Cheating after you are at your goal and you want to maintain it."

Okay, yeah, let's talk about this. Two thumbs way up.

"During the descent to her goal weight, I like a woman to be extremely focused and to have a militarian mind-set of plowing, plodding, and keeping her nose to the grindstone. Some women do better if they do not cheat at all until they get to their Goal A weight. No bread. No alcohol. No dessert. But other women do better if they can have a little pleasure along the way. So if a woman wants one cheat item a week, I allow it. One cheat item would be two glasses of wine, two pieces of bread, or one dessert."

That is not cheating. That is merely a drop in the bucket. Dang, I thought I was going to get more than that. That is diddly-squat.

"After a woman reaches her goal weight," he says, "she can maintain her weight by allowing two to three cheat items a week. Since she is weighing every day, she will not be surprised by a five-pound weight gain. This is how wise women maintain their skinny bodies after they get to their goal weights: they weight every day, stay on this healthy program, and add back a little starch or sweet to see how much their bodies will allow before they rebel and gain back a couple pounds. Some women can have three or four cheat items a week. But what women must understand is there is *never a return to what was before.* Never will they be able to stray far from these principles if they want to maintain their skinniness. Skinny women maintain their skinniness by diligently watching and managing what they put into their mouths and how much they move their bodies the rest of their lives."

The rest of my life? Dang.

"There is a fantasy that after one gets to her goal weight," he says, "then she can begin to eat as she did before. Not a chance. That way of eating whatever and whenever is gone for good. You will allow yourself Planned Cheats, and you will not 'fall into' them. The diligence and watchdog approach must never be abandoned. It is now a permanent feature in your life."

This is stupid to admit, but somehow I was hoping that eventually, I could go back to eating on demand, whatever and whenever. I know it is ludicrous, but that is what I really want, so that is what I somehow allowed myself to think on a deep, subconscious level. I still possess a little insanity thinking about food.

"Genie, the fact that I will never be able to go back to my old friend, Trash Food, is hurtful to think about," I say.

"Did you hear yourself?" he asks. "You called Trash Food your friend. Jackie, Trash Food was your enemy. It ruined your life. It made you fat and gave you constant discouragement. You have to remember that healthy food is your friend, and Trash Food is your archenemy."

How long have I been in this program? And my brain still defaults to wanting and longing for Trash Food? I am not ready for *Skinny School* to be over! Not by a long shot.

"I have left you a recipe of Genie Crab-Stuffed Shrimp in your fridge," he says and disappears. My mind is still trying to get itself to embrace his words, *the rest of your life*, but I hear Zach hang up the phone, and I decide to think about the Genie's talk later.

Zach and I get back in his car. Glancing at him, I notice how his jeans lock around his worked-out quads and his shirt falls into his flat six-pack abs. I smell him. This is intoxicating for me. Ms. Runner-Up is some lucky girl. Zach's phone rings, and it is his mother. "Take it," I encourage him. Zach's phone is routed through the speakers on his car, so I can hear the whole conversation. "Hi, honey," the cheerful voice begins. "I hate to bother you, but your dad is out of town, and my car will not start. I have bridge club at two, and I was wondering how you felt about giving me a jump. Are you busy?"

"Jackie is with me," he says. "I need to take her home, and that is around thirty minutes away, so it will be an hour before I get there."

"Where does she live?" I ask.

"A few miles from here," he says.

"That is crazy for you to drive me home first," I say. "Let's just run by now."

His mother obviously heard our entire conversation and says, "I would love to meet Jackie, since you say such wonderful things about her."

I wonder what Zach has said about me. But quickly, I realize he has told her that I am a crackerjack assistant who can write briefs. Duh. I am a basket case, still hoping for a few crumbs from Zach.

Zach glances at me, and I nod that I really am okay with stopping.

Zach turns around, and in about ten minutes, we pull up to a palace. I mean a real storybook palace. This is old money right here. Very old money.

Mrs. Boltz is tall but very slim. She has on stone-colored jeans with a turquoise shirt. Her red hair is cut in a bob and has a little edgy look to it for someone who is obviously in her late fifties. Her skin is smooth. I wonder if she has had any work done—I am pretty sure she has. She has a classy and conservative look, as if she has had a maid and a cook all her life. Her teeth are white, and her nails have an obviously fresh French manicure. Her warmth is instantaneous as she shakes my hand. She kisses Zach on the cheek and says, "You have a pretty assistant, Zach."

Immediately I feel accepted and comfortable in the presence of this elegant lady.

There is a little white dog named Ellie yapping and running around the kitchen, which Mrs. Boltz talks to as if it were a grandchild. I play with Ellie while Mrs. Boltz and Zach jump the battery in her car. When they walk back in the kitchen, Mrs. Boltz begins to thank Zach profusely for stopping by, telling him she knows how busy he is and how much she appreciates this. Her vivaciousness and energy are contagious. I am pretty sure Zach inherited his father's personality.

Mrs. Boltz says to Zach, "Is this the assistant who can write briefs, Zach?"

"Right here in the flesh, the one and only," he says, glancing at me with a slight grin.

"How do you like working for my son?" she asks.

I tell Zach's mom about how he focuses and does not take breaks. I tell her how he seems all business, but I hear him giving part of his fee to poor clients. Mrs. Boltz and I laugh together as she realizes how I have her son figured out.

It is like a little secret society that has immediately developed between the two of us: we both get Zach Boltz. I can feel her approval of me.

"Where did you get your brains, dear? From your mother or your father?" she asks.

"I am not sure how many brains I have," I lie to appear modest, "but I am definitely a cross between the two. My dad is the creative one, but my mom was the logical thinker." Zach told me on the ride here that his mom has a PhD in clinical psychology. I feel like I might now be entering therapy.

"Zach says you are considering going to law school, Jackie," Mrs. Boltz says.

"I was," I answer, "but now instead I may try to figure out how to support myself so I can write."

Zach already knows this. He glances over at me and our eyes meet.

"Jackie is dating Thomas Fleetwood, Mom," Zach says.

"Oh! I know him," Mrs. Boltz says. "Such a nice young man! As adorable as you are—I am not surprised."

I do not know why she thinks I am adorable. I am just a middle-class American girl.

"Zach, you need to find someone as adorable as Jackie to date. Does she have a sister?" she says and laughs.

"Yes," he replies, "but they are all married."

I cannot quite describe how I feel at this moment. Me, an ex-chubby but now slim, standing in Zach Boltz's mother's kitchen, and she is telling me how adorable I am and telling Zach to find someone as cute as me to date. Why, six months ago, this woman would never have said this to fat Jackie. Weight loss changes how I feel about myself, and as much as I hate to admit this, it changes how others feel about me, too.

Zach begins to leave, and his mother thanks him again for coming by.

"Jackie, I hope to see more of you. My, what a delightful girl you are!" And she hugs me. Zach and I both get back in his car.

"My mom was crazy about you," he says.

"Well, what does your mom think about Ms. Runner-Up?" I ask.

Zach looks at me with surprise on his face. "She hasn't met her," he says.

"She hasn't met her?" I ask. "I thought she moved here."

"She did," he answers.

"So I'm surprised your mom hasn't met her," I say.

"I don't know why. I haven't seen her since New Year's Eve, Jack."

Shocked. That is what I am. Stunned. "I assumed you were dating," I say.

"Dating?" He laughs. "We aren't dating. She isn't my type."

Again, I am bewildered. I assumed they were planning a wedding.

"Not your type?" I ask, astounded.

"Not my type," he says.

"How could a blue-blooded, orphan-loving, Miss Runner-Up not be your type, Zach?"

He laughs again. "So you think you have me figured out, do you? Jack, obviously, you don't."

My text beeps, and it is Thomas.

"Now there is a nice guy," Zach says. "How are things going with Thomas?"

"Okay, I guess," I respond. But I cannot think straight. All this time, I thought Zach was dating Ms. Runner-Up. This new information is mind-boggling.

Zach drops me off at my apartment, and I get ready for my tennis date, who sure does talk a lot.

Lesson 23

The Genie Departs

Monday, January 26   *Weight: 135*   *Pounds lost: 40*   *Still to go: 5*

Thomas and I hung out most of the weekend. However, all I could think about was that Ms. Runner-Up is not Zach's type and that they are not dating. I am still stunned. Usually, I am so good at reading people and situations, but my assumptions were certainly wrong this time.

Thomas is driving to Murfreesboro this morning, a city about thirty minutes away, for a deposition, but he should be back after lunch. I am not very excited about Thomas anymore. His constant chattering has become annoying to me.

Because Eva is sick today, I drive to the post office to pick up some packages that could not be delivered over the weekend. **In transit, my dear Middle Eastern friend appears in my passenger seat.** I have developed a granddaughterly affection for my sage counselor.

"Young Jackie, congratulations on your weight loss. You were 135 pounds this morning!" the Genie says. "And the wonderful thing is you now know how to stay at this weight forever. No more fad diets or regaining the weight."

"Being thin is a pleasure that far surpasses any sacrifice I have made in not eating Trash Food," I say. "What is especially wonderful is the new degree of self-forgetfulness. My weight is no longer the central issue in my life."

Confessing that last statement is not comfortable, as I know it reveals a certain degree of previous shallowness. But it is, at least, honest.

"That is a common remark of the women I have helped in *Skinny School*, Young Jackie. I too am happy about your newfound emotional freedom."

"What lesson do you have today?" I ask. My mind is still in a bit of a tizzy over Zach not dating Ms. Runner-Up, as well as worrying about what to do with Thomas, but I am up for another lesson. I absolutely *love* being thin. Last weekend, I bought a pair of European size twenty-nine Lucky jeans! Woo-hoo!

"*Skinny School* lessons are officially over," the Genie says. "Today we will have a final review."

Gulp...uh...what? Over? Over? "I'm not ready for *Skinny School* to be over, Genie. I still have five pounds to lose." If I got the wish and the Genie, shouldn't I be the one to say when this class is over?

"You now know all the secrets, and you do not need me anymore. Therefore, I will review the main tenets of *Skinny School* and depart. First, we will make our last list, List Ten, in your Ruby Journal and call it 'Important Thoughts That Retrain My Brain.' You already have many thoughts in your Ruby Journal, but I want you to write down anything from today's review that you feel would be helpful in retraining your brain how to think."

My brain has been washed with much new thought in *Skinny School*, for sure, but the default mode is still set to listen to my Demanding Child and her incessant desire for using food for soothing and entertainment. At least I know I must feed my Sane Adult with the right thought, or I will cave in to my strong lower impulses.

"Women invariably refuse to read their Ruby Journals as often as I want them to," he says, "but just know that the women who have the most success in retraining their brains in how to think correctly about eating and exercise *are the ones who override their previous neural pathways and thought patterns* by being faithful in doing this daily reading. Your prior thinking is like a strong undertow, and to counteract that powerful force, you must read your Ruby Journal frequently."

He is not kidding when he describes my prior thinking as a strong undertow.

"*Skinny School* women collect good thought," he says, "like some people collect rare paintings or fine sculptures. They know that thinking the right thoughts is the ticket to skinniness."

The impact of daily reading my Ruby Journal is inestimable.

"One reason why women are able to choose against Trash Food," he reminds me, "is they realize being thin and fit is simply one of the greatest pleasures women experience. Therefore, giving up a short-lived taste experience loses its pull to something that is ultimately much more satisfying and fulfilling."

I can now agree with that sentence. Thinking back over the past few months, I again realize I do not miss the sugar or carbs in comparison with how much I enjoy my new size.

"Even before a woman gets to her goal," he says, "she experiences joy and freedom when she stays on her program as eating clean makes her feel great, physically and emotionally. The self-mastery itself feels invigorating. However, when a woman goes off her plan, she experiences discouragement and self-incrimination."

Clean eating is invigorating; eating Trash Food stinks. Check.

"Wise women manage their eating and exercise like they do their hair or brushing their teeth. It is a nonnegotiable part of every day."

Who can believe that every morning I think about what I am going to eat that day and when I am going to exercise?

"Restricting your food is *not* about deprivation," he says. "Instead, it is about going after something you want more. Yes, *Skinny School* students are definitely giving up immediate pleasure by giving up Trash Food, but they are obtaining a much higher pleasure, thinness! And by choosing well today, a wise woman is choosing against the inevitable discouragement of tomorrow that comes with going off her plan. Wise women stick to their plans because they remember how terrible they feel when they don't."

Ah, yes. The inevitable down-and-depressed mood that I know all too well.

"Wise women know that they, like all women, will have low moods," he says. "They keep their Ruby Journal handy, so they can readily access their motivational readings. Then they make some delicious herbal tea and open up their Quart Bags."

He forgot to mention soup! Quart Bags and soup!

"When a *Skinny School* woman sees others eating Trash Food, she does not feel sorry for herself that she does not get any," he says. "She rejoices that she is going to have a thin body and actually feels sorry for these women who are still in bondage to Trash Food. The *Skinny School* woman knows there is pleasure in Trash Food but remembers the higher pleasure in having a skinny tush."

My tush is now a size six. Size *six*!

"Champions battle for their goals," he says. "They are wildly proactive to reach their goals instead of giving some piddly-wink, two-bit effort. They choose *colossal, mammoth effort* to reach their goals."

The old me gave a piddly-wink effort but not the new me. I can almost hear the *Rocky* overture playing.

"Successful *Skinny School* women see all food," he says, "as a choice either for thinness, well-being, health, confidence, joy, and self-mastery *or* for frumpiness, discouragement, and low health."

Hey! No frump here anymore.

"*Skinny School* women begin to see their food choices as either making them fit, lean, emotionally free, and happy, *or* frumpy, upset, envious, and down. Choosing what you eat is actually a choice for how you will experience life."

That is a pretty crazy, over-the-top comment, but after being upset with being fat for thirteen years, I know he is right.

"There will be no permanent progress in *Skinny School*," he says, "until a woman understands that sugars and starches must be replaced with proteins, good fats, and vegetables. This new eating habit will get rid of cravings and subsequent feelings of insanity."

Giving up sugar and starches for self-soothing and entertainment has been the hardest part of this program, but I have done it. I have really done it.

"Wise women realize how much they care that they live their one, short life on earth in a small body, and they make choices all day long so that is true," he says. "Being overweight is not an option for wise women. Exercise is not an option. Trash Food is not a part of their world."

It seems hard to believe that Trash Food is not a part of my world anymore, but it truly isn't.

"*Skinny School* women find great delight in their food," he says. "They wait until they are hungry, and then have gorgeous, healthy food available. They never indulge in self-pity. They exalt in feeding their bodies the Creator's beautiful, delicious food. Trash Food and eating when one is not hungry are actually the killers of dreams, not the delights they pretend to be. Instead, restricting your food is the high, true pleasure. I have told you before that initially, women see key lime pie as zest, delight, stimulation, color, and life. But instead, the best way to think about key lime pie is as the destroyer of your dreams and a two-minute taste experience that messes up your health, since sugar and refined carbs are bad for you. Eating key lime pie is an invitation to be overweight, which is keeping you from one of your current Top Four Life Goals. Key lime pie is not your friend but an enemy that is disguising itself in a two-minute taste experience."

Yes, an enemy in disguise. True, very true.

"A helpful secret is to not desire Trash Food," he says. "When you see that the sugar in cakes and cookies wrecks your health, your weight, your emotional freedom, your blood, then you can begin to *not* desire it and see it for the monster it is."

Me seeing sugar as a monster—ha-ha, funny.

"I want to remind you where Champions separate from the average: it is in planning and prepping. This work is the winner's edge," he reminds me.

No longer do I whine about the planning and prepping anymore; it is now part of my daily schedule.

"Planning and prepping food is an expected part of a wise woman's schedule. Fail to plan, then plan to fail"

That reminds me, I need to go to the grocery store. I run out of vegetables so quickly.

"Wise women daily preplan their meals, having the necessary food in the house," he says. "They do not begrudge the work, as these behaviors take them where they want to go, adding more Willpower Points to their day."

Grocery shopping is now a staple in the week's activities. Honestly, I do not even mind washing and prepping veggies anymore; the habit is now ingrained.

"In fact, *Skinny School* women do not begrudge the many aspects of the work it is to be thin: the planning, shopping, prepping, cooking, exercising, and writing in the Ruby Journal. They understand that their current Top Four Life Goals should take some effort, and they are happy to do these behaviors. They realize that this investment of time and energy will never go completely away. They make time in their days for these habits for the rest of their lives."

Getting my mind around *the rest of my life* has been a little hard to do, but I think I'm finally there.

"Wise women love eating small meals when they are hungry and stopping before they are full," he says. "They exalt in this self-control, as it gives them one of their current Top Four Life Goals. Their strictness and austerity gives them a feeling of *pleasure, not deprivation*. They know this is one of the best ways in the world they can take care of themselves. They also know when they take care of themselves, they will then have more energy *to take care of others*."

Demanding Child has tried to convince me that this program is too self-focused so she could eat right away, but the truth is, I have more energy now to give to others.

"Just like everyone else, *Skinny School* students want a snack before bedtime, but when they are not truly hungry, they get something calorie free and soothing to drink instead. These women will soon be asleep—and will be happy in the morning that they did not eat."

I used to think ice cream helped me sleep.

"Wise women portion out their foods," he says. "Of course, *they could always eat more*, but they eat just enough *to kill hunger. Enough is as good as a feast,* they constantly tell themselves. They eat slowly and wait for twenty minutes so the stomach can tell the brain they have had enough."

Stopping at a five is *still* a very difficult thing to do. Food can be so yummy!

"Large quantities of even healthy food are not desirable," he says. "What is desirable is thinness, and to achieve thinness, women must eat small amounts of healthy food. *Skinny School* students are never hungry, though. They eat when they are truly physically hungry."

Well, thank goodness. I could not do this school if I had to be hungry.

"*Skinny School* women repeatedly are grateful for the emotional freedom they experience when they stick to their plans. They realize that eating Trash Food—or eating when they are not hungry—will diminish this joy."

Emotional freedom is amazing. It is something I now have more of than I have ever had before.

"The daily pull of the Demanding Child will never go away," he says, "so *Skinny School* women are always on watch for her conniving schemes to eat in ways that are not in line with the Sane Adult's true goals. Even though the Demanding Child will always be whiney and demanding, you do not have to give in to her. You enable your Sane Adult to overrule the incessant drumbeat of the Demanding Child by frequently reading your Ruby Journal."

I am doing better. Yes, much better.

"The idea of trying to have both Trash Food and thinness must be confronted. Give up Trash Food until you are at Goal A. Yes, there is sacrifice in *Skinny School*, but that is how life works: sacrifice something deemed *good* to get something actually *better*."

Definitely, I have made great strides in giving up the idea of having *both*.

"A *Skinny School* woman does not waste time arguing with herself about what she will eat. The daily debate about what she will eat or whether she will exercise is over. She chooses what is best for herself *long-term*, not what is most pleasant *now*."

Who can believe I eat apple slices instead of popcorn while watching a movie?

"Women who have rejected the pleas of their Demanding Child and who are now thin never say, 'I regret all the planning, shopping, tracking, prepping, waiting, and cooking.' They say they are absolutely, positively thrilled with their new lives. However, the women who give in to their Demanding Child still feel discouraged and have regret."

I know discouragement. I know regret.

"Wise women realize they are in control of their eating, and their eating is not in control of them," he says. "*Skinny School* students realize they choose to be in shape or overweight by *what they eat, how much they eat, and how much they move*. Although they love desserts *like everyone else*, they avoid them because they do not get them what they really want most. They work hard to find other means of self-soothing and stimulation."

Not perfect by a long shot, but wow, what an improvement I am from my past days!

"Emotional eating must be confronted, and substitute behaviors, such as taking a bath, calling a friend, taking a walk, chomping down on the Quart Bags or a cup of soup, reading a book or a magazine, listening to music or a sermon, drawing a picture, etcetera, must be learned."

Walking definitely makes me feel better.

"Exercise is often difficult in the moment, but it must be done," he continues. "There is simply no other way to stay healthy. Wise women *push through their uncomfortable, everyday resistance to exercise.* Many women add great music to their workouts. Exercise is a part of most days, and *Skinny School* students realize they do not truly feel great about a day without exercise."

As much as I still hate to exercise, I do feel fabulous when I am through and guilty if I skip it. I need to star that thought in my Ruby Journal.

"*Skinny School* women eventually become addicted to exercise in a good way," he says, "knowing the vast benefits they receive from exercise. They see exercise as a nonnegotiable part of most days. They work hard to find ways to enjoy exercise. They know they will battle internal resistance—Demanding Child—most days, but they find a way to push past this hurdle."

Battling internal resistance to exercise is *every* day, not most days.

"Wise women know who they hang around influences their eating. Friends and family who love and esteem Trash Food will tempt you to eat it," he says. "Friends and family who eat the Creator's food encourage you to eat on your program."

I must remember to be on guard against this.

"Wise *Skinny School* women know that their choosing mechanisms are not at their best at night when they are tired. Therefore, they pay extra attention to their nighttime behaviors. The magnetic, powerful pull for immediate gratification is only overcome by a diligent effort to remind your Sane Adult what you really want, so wise women redouble their efforts at night."

Having good herbal teas available at night has been a lifesaver.

"Wise women never blame anyone else for their weight issues," he says. "They know that ultimately only they are in charge of their choices. They do not allow anyone to push food on them. They are polite but still say, 'no, thank you.'"

If I can withstand Eva's food pushing, I can withstand anyone's.

"*Skinny School* graduates have a mind-set about how they eat and how they exercise and even have rules for Planned Cheating. Wise women do not use food to change the way they feel. They use food for nutrition and hunger. They want to live in a thin body, so they live a certain way, every day, for the rest of their lives. They work hard at finding stimulation, entertainment, and self-soothing in other areas besides food."

That is a growth in process, learning how to handle my emotions without eating them down. The Quart Bags have been an important tool in my toolkit, as have soups.

"Successful women in *Skinny School* know that no one is coming on a white horse to rescue them," he says, "so they take full responsibility for their eating, blaming no one and nothing but themselves."

Earlier, I wanted to blame some of my eating on Eva's annoying personality.

"Alcohol is strictly quarantined if you are going to drink it at all, as alcohol slows down the metabolism," he says.

At least that is one problem I do not have. Now, thinking of Chloe, that is another story. I think she had three glasses of wine one night during Christmas. Eek!

"Retraining the brain *cannot* be done in a day or even a month," he says. *Skinny School* women daily wash their brains with correct new thought for months."

The magazines at the checkout at the grocery store promise results in two weeks. Bogus stuff.

"Strong self-discipline, willpower, and strictness take you to new heights of enjoyment. Self-mastery has a unique joy."

Ha-ha, who can believe I would ever say I love self-discipline?

"*Self-restraint* is the virtue, not *indulgence*. It is absurd to think otherwise," he says. "Don't wish for skinniness; work for it. Champions expect their goals to be inconvenient and so do not whine about them."

Indulgence was the sought-after experience for so long.

"Wise women get weighed every day of their lives. They know they will have a couple pounds of water that will make their weight vary, but by weighing every day, they make themselves face the truth. Foodsters need to weigh daily."

Is *foodsters* a cuss word for fat chicks?

"So now it is time to depart, Young Jackie," he says. "Your wish to be skinny has been granted."

It is true. The keys to the kingdom of thinness have been given to me. I will never get over my gratitude for the information that will forever keep me out of the Food Dungeon where I was chained to chubbiness.

"Remember the best way to seal these truths in your heart is to teach them," he says. "Gather together a few friends and share these truths with them. Over a period of a few months, your brain will further cement the ideas as you explain them to others."

Finally, I am ready to gather a few friends and begin. I should have done this months earlier.

"It is now time for you to give me to someone else who could use some help from a Genie," he says.

I think of my Ashley, my BFF from college who repeatedly struggles with severe discouragement and who could use a *Happy School*. I will have to think about who to give the Genie to.

"You have been one of my favorite students ever," he says, and with that last smile, the Genie disappears.

With the Genie leaving me for good, I am pretty emotionally wiped out. Being on my own is scary. I hope I am ready.

After returning from the post office, I try to get focused on my day's work but have much difficulty. It is around eleven o'clock, and I hear some yelling from the foyer, which is around twenty yards away. Zach quickly comes out of his office and glances down the hall to see what is going on. Attorney Simpson's office is on the other side of the foyer, and the yelling seems to be moving in that direction.

After surveying what is happening in the foyer, Zach turns to me and says, "Jack, I want you to call nine-one-one right now, and then get under your desk. There is a man with a gun in the foyer. Then no matter what—do you hear me, no matter what—do not get up until the police arrive." And with that, he walks down the hall toward the foyer.

The terror I feel cannot be described. Time stands still. Though I feel frozen like an ice statue, I will my fingers to bring my phone to my eyes and punch in nine-one-one, and somehow my fingers move. Nine. One. One. I wait. The rings are so long. I never knew a ring could last so long. And the space between the rings is very long. A ring again. Another long space. I hear yelling and screaming from down the hall. I hear the angry voice of one of our clients, Mr. Pierce. And finally, the most beautiful voice I have ever heard speaks, "Nine-one-one, what is your emergency?"

Again, I will my voice to speak, but I do not even sound like myself. "There is a...man...with a gun...here. Please...send...help." And I start blurting out the address. I am whispering but being very careful to speak plainly. My body feels like I was just jolted with an electric current and I am a hot wire, myself. I am a combination of paralyzed and jolted with electric current. I feel more like a machine than a human.

I pray. I pray with a pleading that I have never prayed with before.

I hear a gunshot. My stomach falls to the ground.

"I've got it. I've got the gun. Hold him, Zach. Hold him," I hear Attorney Simpson's voice boom from down the hall.

I'm not sure what happened, but Zach is not shot and must have Mr. Pierce in some sort of hold. And Attorney Simpson has the gun. My body still feels the shock of the crisis, but I have hopes they have subdued the man without any harm. I hear sirens coming in the distance. As the sirens become closer, I count the long seconds. I listen to hear every sound from down the hall, but the approaching sirens drown out all noise.

The police rush in the front door, and I hear Zach's calm voice tell the officers what happened. Zach is okay. Zach is not hurt. The tears start flowing down my face in uncontrollable streams. Getting up, I run down the hall, past the foyer, and into Attorney Simpson's office where the entire episode happened. Zach sees me as I rush in. Instinctively, I know that I am to rush to him. His eyes do not leave me as I approach, and his arms open to embrace me before I am halfway to him. I am sobbing now, and his arms comfort me like I am a little child.

"I was so afraid, Zach," I sob.

"I know. But you are safe, now, Jack. You are safe. That is what I prayed… that you would be safe." His arms are still holding me tightly, not even beginning to let go. The fear of the previous moments now coupled with Zach's strong arms around me make me feel alive in a way that I can never remember feeling. Life, so precious, so fragile.

He slowly lets go of his strong hold on me and gazes into my eyes. "You are safe now, Jack." And again, he says, "That is all I kept thinking about, that I wanted you to be safe."

I cannot believe he is saying this. His eyes are moist, but he regains control immediately. Mr. Pierce is ushered out, and the officers want to talk to Zach.

Zach is giving a play-by-play of the account, and Attorney Simpson interrupts. "This boy is a hero. I was sitting at my desk, and Pierce comes in and points a gun at my face. Zach diverts his attention, knocks the gun out of his hand, and it goes off. Then this fine young man apprehends him while I scramble to get the gun. Zach Boltz is a hero, I tell you, a hero."

The police want to question Zach some more, staying another thirty minutes.

After the police leave, Zach and I slowly and silently walk back toward our offices. We walk with slow steps, obviously with thoughts of what could have happened weighing on both of us. Zach starts to go into his office and turns to me. "Jack, come in here a second, please."

As I walk into his office, he closes the door behind me. I turn to look at him to see what is going on. "I need to talk to you about something," Zach says.

The emotion of the moment still has me shaking. I hope he does not want to talk about any upcoming briefs that need to be written.

"I know you are dating Thomas, but when I saw Mr. Pierce with that gun, I said to myself, 'Zach, if you die, you will never get to tell Jack you love her.'"

Did he say *tell* Jack *you love her*? *Jack*, as in me? I pause and do not say anything, and neither does he. Finally I speak.

"Is the *Jack* you are talking about *me*?" I need to be sure.

He thinks that comment is hilarious. "Yes, you are the Jack I am talking about," he says, and he laughs again.

It was not a bad question. What if there was another Jack?

"When Mr. Pierce was standing there with the gun," Zach says, "our future passed before my eyes: our marriage, our home, our lake house..."

I burst out laughing when he says *lake house*. I am faint. Thomas must have just arrived back from Murfreesboro, and I can hear him out in the hall calling for me. I act like I don't hear him.

Zach continues to stand still, staring at me with his gray-green eyes.

"Marry someone you can't live without," he says. "I can't live without you, Jack."

"You can't?" I ask, still not believing this moment.

"You know Thomas is not right for you, don't you?" he asks.

"I...I admit it. He...is...not," I somehow say.

"And you know we are supposed to be together, right?" he asks.

My brain is spinning. Before I know what is happening, Zach gathers me in his arms and kisses me like I have only seen kisses in the movies. Zach Boltz is kissing me. This is better than *You've Got Mail* and *Sleepless in Seattle* combined.

"We are supposed to be together, and you know it," he says. "We will get married soon, and you will not have to work. You can stay home, write your novel, and take care of our six kids."

Again I burst out laughing when he says *six kids*. I start crying, too, all at the same time. Prince Charming is in love with Middle-Class Jackie. This is a real-life picture of when Prince Charming puts the shoe on servant-girl Cinderella's foot.

Thomas is loudly calling for me now. I dry my face and try to get myself together.

"Jack, I want you to break up with Thomas as soon as you can," Zach says. I can't talk, but I shake my head yes.

"I'll be over at six tonight, and then we'll go to dinner and discuss our next seventy years together." When he says *seventy years*, I burst out crying all over again. Drying my face one more time, I start to go out in the hall as Thomas's calls for me are getting louder and louder.

"One more thing, Jack," Zach says. I turn around.

"I have loved you for months. I think I first realized it in September, the night we ate dinner with Beth and Richard and I took you home." He starts grinning that grin of his as he continues, "You were so scared that I thought you had set it up and that I was going to think you were pursuing me. You must have said three times that you got invited at the last minute."

He saw through that?

He grins again, "You were so beautiful in the candlelight that night. I remember thinking, 'Here is a girl who is smart, pretty, and funny.' Yes, I think I started falling in love with you that night."

September? I still weighed 165 pounds back then! I was a tub. He started falling in love with me then?

I don't tell him that I think I fell in love with him the first moment I met him, the moment he interviewed me to be his assistant. He does not need to know that...until after the wedding.

"And remember at the skating rink in November," he continues, "when we were talking about the few moments when I did not feel lonely? I realized right then that I did not feel lonely when I was with you."

That was the night of the wreck when he and Rachel broke up. I was 147 pounds then. I am such an idiot. The man of my dreams just told me loves me and wants to marry me, and I am thinking about my weight. I am a nutcase.

Zach Boltz loves me. And I know how to be skinny the rest of my life. I'm afraid I might explode, I'm so happy.

Walking into the hall, I see Thomas, and he tries to hug me. We walk outside, and I tell him that when I was staring death in the face, I realized that he and I were not right for each other. He doesn't like it, but what is he going to say? I don't mention Zach. One thing at a time.

Attorney Simpson closes the office early as everyone is shell-shocked. I drive home, trying to take in the day's events. Am I really the girl Zach Boltz wants to spend the rest of his life with? Me? Ordinary me?

I weighed 135 pounds this morning, and even though ideally, I would like to lose five more pounds, I feel marvelously thin. I have a new camel skirt to wear to dinner tonight that is two inches above my knees, along with some great-looking brown suede boots. Ha-ha—I am a skinny girl! I am a skinny girl who has the secrets to being thin forever. And now, I am going to live my skinny life with the man of my dreams!

When that brown package with the Genie arrived on my doorstep last August, I was in the pit, the deep, dark pit of being locked in a Food Dungeon. Life stunk, and I had no idea how to escape. But now, just a few short months later, I have acquired two of my current Top Four Life Goals! Me, plain ole Jackie! The chubby girl in high school.

At this moment, I love life. I absolutely love it. And to think that I used to let food and my Demanding Child rule my life. Ha!

Thank you, Genie. From the bottom of my heart, thank you, thank you, thank you. You rock to the moon and back.

Wow. Life is awesome.

Epilogue
Eight Years Later

Zach and Jackie currently have three kids, although Zach is still pressing for more. Even during her pregnancies, Jackie kept her weight down and got back to 132 pounds eight weeks after each childbirth. She has just completed her second novel, and a large national publisher is interested in acquiring the rights to both of her books. Jackie loves her skinniness and frequently has groups of women meet in her home, where she teaches them the secrets in *Skinny School*. Jackie still *ditches, plans, tracks, preps, makes Quart Bags, schedules her exercise, writes in her Ruby Journal, keeps a clean environment, and waits until she is physically hungry to eat.* Last weekend, Zach and Jackie put a contract down on a lake house.

Appendix A

The Ruby Journal Lists

List 1: My Top Four Life Goals

List 2: My Goal Weights: A, B, and Scream Zone

List 3: Master Options List

List 4: Tracking Sheet for Hunger/Hunger Scale

List 5: Repeated Schemes My Demanding Child Uses

List 6: Pleasures and Comforts in Life besides Food

List 7: Benefits of Exercise

List 8: What Exercise Will I Do?

List 9: Ways to Relax, Replenish, and Reward Myself besides Food

List 10: Important Thoughts That Retrain My Brain

You can download free pages to make your Ruby Journal at JulieNGordon.com.

Appendix B

The Nine Nonnegotiables of Skinny School

1. I expect to work hard like a Champion to retrain my mind since this is a Top Four Life Goal.

2. Ditching sweets and starches is not optional if I want to overhaul my metabolism.

3. Planning and prepping are the secrets that Champions use to conquer goals. I must make daily Quart Bags and I must track my food *as I eat it.*

4. Hunger is my friend, and waiting until I am truly hungry and quitting before I am full are nonnegotiable. Tracking my hunger is imperative and will expose how I deceive myself with wanting to eat for self-soothing and entertainment.

5. By listing the schemes of Demanding Child in my Ruby Journal and accessing how my Sane Adult really feels, I can dismantle my Demanding Child's tricks, one by one.

6. Failure can be useful, if I will evaluate it and learn from it.

7. Finding substitutes for soothing and entertaining myself besides food is imperative.

8. A clean environment, one without Trash Food, is crucial to reduce temptation.

9. Daily I will face resistance to exercise, and probably will forever. Therefore, I must plan and prep like Champions do to accomplish their Top Four Life Goals.

Appendix C
List of Genie Recipes

All recipes are online at JulieNGordon.com.

Lesson 1: Genie Meatballs

Lesson 2: Genie Taco Salad

Lesson 3: Genie Chicken Vegetable Soup

Lesson 4: Genie Salmon

Lesson 5: Genie Quiche

Lesson 6: Genie Almond-Flour Fried Chicken

Lesson 7: Genie Broiled Chicken Kebabs

Lesson 8: Genie Spinach Salad with Goat Cheese and Bacon with Caesar Dressing

Lesson 9: Genie Vegetable Omelets

Lesson 10: Genie Deviled Eggs

Lesson 11: Genie Deli Turkey Bacon Rollups

Lesson 12: Genie Eggs Benedict with Hollandaise

Lesson 13: Genie Chicken Enchiladas

Lesson 16: Genie Chicken Divan

Lesson 17: Genie Baked Orange Roughy

Lesson 18: Genie Lasagna

Appendix D
Websites of Health Gurus

1. Mercola.com
   Dr. Joseph Mercola is my favorite health expert. He has a daily e-mail that will skyrocket your understanding of health and what to eat. He recommends that people stay under twenty-five or fewer grams of sugar a day. The knowledge you will gain by reading this man's articles will hugely contribute to your health and well-being.

2. MarksDailyApple.com
   Mark Sisson has written a famous Paleo book, *The Primal Blueprint*, which is excellent. This man is changing many lives for the better. He advises his readers that want to lose weight to "stay under fifty carbs a day."

Appendix E

Final Remarks

Dear Reader,

I want you to succeed, but if you cut corners, you will not. I have rewritten again some of the main tenets of *Skinny School*. Do not leave anything to chance! Remember, it is a sowing and reaping world.

To Your Goal A,

Julie Gordon

1. You have to sincerely want to be thin to do the hard work of changing how you think (Lesson 1). If you don't care about being thin, then this program will be too much work. *Sincere, heart-felt values and goals drive and create motivation and discipline,* not the other way around. Getting in touch with what you truly care about is the foundational *must* of this program…and reminding yourself of that daily. The *lessons in* Skinny School *are how you permanently change* your mind about food and eating. But if you won't do the work the Genie commands, then you must learn to be content with being overweight (or those other awful words, *frumpy* and *fat*.)

2. Three things determine if you are thin:
   What you eat (Lesson 2)

How much you eat (Lesson 4)

How much you move (Lesson 9)

But remember, *the mind chooses* all three of those components, so reprogramming the brain is key!

3. Since you have an issue with food, you must do the work to preplan and preprep (Lesson 3). Human willpower will fail you, so you must make provisions to protect yourself (Sane Adult) from yourself (Demanding Child). Quart Bags are lifesavers!

4. *Do* not *fear failure*, and *do* not *throw this program out the window* when you fail. Mark this down: you will fail! Instead, when you fail, evaluate it, learn from it, write about it in your Ruby Journal, and get back on the bus immediately. *How you handle failure will largely determine your success.* You must not get discouraged when you fail but know that failure is part of *any Champion's program* to conquer a problem. Learn that failure holds the hidden secrets to overcoming your obstacle—if you will evaluate it. If you lose your way, remember the Miraculous Threesome: Ditch, Plan, Wait!

5. Repetition is the key to learning, so read and reread and reread the Genie portions. Your mind's thinking is like a schoolyard path that is made by constant use. We are going to close down the old path and make a new path for the school children. Eventually, the old path will regrow grass, and the new path will be made. This is the way your brain works. But it takes time, and you must repeatedly bathe your mind with the new thought. That is why this is a twenty-three-week program. Honestly, reading the Genie portion one time is *not nearly enough*. I expect my students to read and reread the Genie portions until the Genie's teaching becomes their go-to thought about food and eating. If you follow this program as I lay it out, you eventually will be able to look at dessert (carbs, sugar, etc.) and because of your new mind-set, you will be able to choose to not have it. This is the magic of the program, being able to choose to eat for nutrition and hunger, not for self-soothing or entertainment!

6. When I tell people that *Skinny School* graduates who have reached their Goal A weight *still* make Quart Bags, *still* plan their exercise, *still* keep a clean environment, *still* ditch sugar and starches, many are surprised. Most people have a mind-set that once you reach your goal weight, you can revert to prior behaviors. Heavens, no. Although all *Skinny School* graduates still have a very ornery and seductive Demanding Child, they keep her in check with daily disciplines. Friends, this program will give you back the life that being fat has stolen.

7. The recipes for "eating Paleo" are abundant on the Internet. Be sure to try new recipes. (You will need to decide whether you can have dairy products, such as cheese, Greek yogurt, etc.)

8. Life is not about being skinny; it is about God filling you with Himself so you can do His will (i.e., *faith expressing itself through love*, Galatians 5:6). But the Enemy uses Trash Food in a woman's life to keep her self-focused...away from freedom and joy. But you now have a ticket to get out of the Food Dungeon, the Miraculous Threesome: Ditch, Plan, Wait. Yay!

9. Humans are group creatures. Whom we have coffee with determines, to a large extent, how we think. Be intentional and use this concept to help you quantumly change how you think about food. Gather three to five like-minded friends who also want to change how they think about food. Meet weekly for twenty-three weeks, follow the Group Reading Guide (Appendix F), and sign up for the free twenty-three-week *Skinny School Online* lessons (go to JulieNGordon.com for more information). Take twenty-three weeks to conquer this very hurtful issue in your life. And then with the abundance of new energy you will gain once you overcome your problem with food and eating, use your gifts to *restore a broken world!*

Appendix F
Group Reading Guide

1. To assemble a group, find three to five other highly motivated people. Find women you enjoy. If there is an unpleasant woman in the group, you will not want to meet.

2. Meet weekly for approximately one and a half hours. By discussing one lesson a week, you will meet for twenty-three weeks.

3. Everyone has to agree to fill out her Ruby Journal lists. If a member is not willing to do this, then maybe she should consider being in a group another time.

4. Before the meeting, each group member should highlight the part of the Genie's comments that stands out to her. Then during group time, each person shares why a certain principle or thought stands out to her.

5. Divide the time the group has by how many people are in the group. Everyone should talk for about the same amount of time.

6. Do not give each other unsolicited advice. If a member wants input, she will ask for it.

7. Do not get sidetracked with topics other than the Genie's comments.

8. Share e-mails with each other and write to the group during the week. These e-mails among group members are very encouraging.

After you go through the material once with your first group, it is now time to gather others and *lead them* through this material. Even if you are not at your goal weight, you will have lost many pounds by now. When you are leading others through the study, you will see and understand concepts *you missed the first time*. And when you have to explain this material to others, it further cements the concepts in your mind. Teaching others is the best way to learn anything and also the best way to *permanently reprogram your mind.*

About the Author

Julie Gordon has been happily married to her husband, David, for thirty-one years. Their six children, ages twenty-nine to nineteen, are Elizabeth (married to Trent), Stephen (married to Elaina), Joseph, Jonathan, Benjamin, and Samuel. *Just like you*, love of family is at the top of her list. You can see a picture of Julie's family at her website, JulieNGordon.com.

But next to family, Julie's passion is helping women with their marriages, their eating issues, and their fight for a life of joy in the Lord. Although she has a master's degree in marriage and family counseling, Julie insists that the women in her groups—as well as reading ogles of books—have been her most significant teachers.

On any given day, you can find her writing in her bedroom, cooking (Paleo), going to the gym (still an effort), or texting her kids (even if they don't always text back).

Go to www.JulieNGordon.com for new information, recipes, other books to be released, blogs, and so on. A free twenty-three-week online course, *Skinny School Online*, is now being offered to help you and your group further master the *Skinny School* concepts. Dates of next classes are available at her website.

Search for "*Skinny School*" on Facebook. Enjoy the community. Please post your recipes, pictures of your group, thoughts, and more! Others want to hear what you have to say.

Julie would love to hear your comments. E-mail her at SkinnySchool Online@gmail.com or post a comment addressed to her on Facebook/SkinnySchool.

2 Timothy 1:7: "For the Spirit God…gives us power, love, and self-discipline."

The End

16 Personalities

INFJ

16 Style Types. Facebook

ENTJ
Stubborn al Dominant, Intolerant

Impatient, Arrogant

INFJ
Truth Beauty Purpose

Counselors, Psychologists, Teachers, Social Worker,

Yoga Instructor, Spiritual Leaders.

almost all Mystical.
Yet very Inspiring
and tireless Idealists

Some people need more time to think.

Can intolerable delay to good thinking

commanders.

Poor Handling of Emotions

Cold Ruthless

neither need emotional support

or understand others need for it

Learn
Emotional
Sensitivity

Lack of Sensitivity.

Chicken Weathers'

Though consistant simple actions,
I experience a peaceful pace in my life
allowing for open space of delightful pleasures

Classic - elegant - Sophisticated   <u>Distinct</u>

- balanced - polished

Type 4 Keywords: Bold, Striking, Constant, Still, Firm
Simple <u>Structured</u> class-

Yin 1 - Light, Bright

Black and White

Sleek
Smooth
- Tailored
vapue
well Structured.

X (Captivating)
- classic
Defined
Aligning
- Distinguished / <u>Distinct</u>
- Dramatic
magnificent
majestic
noble
notable
- poised
- Polished
Overtly
Regal

Style Stylist
INFJ
* EN 77
Student Stylist.

Through consistent simple actions,
I experience a peaceful pace in my life
allowing for open spaces of delightful pleasures

Distinct

classic — elegant — sophisticated
— balanced — polished

Type 4 Keywords: Bold, Striking, Constant, Still, Firm
   Simple, Structured, clean

Tab I — Light, Bright

Black and White
★ Captivating
∴ classic
Defined
— Dignified
— Distinguished / Distinct
Dramatic
Magnificent
Majestic
Noble
notable
∴ Poised
∴ Polished
Queenly
— Regal

Sleek
smooth
— Tailored

Vogue
well structured.

Standout Stylist
★ ENTJ

Subtle Stylist
   INFJ

||||||||| |||||||||| |||||||||||
44813019R00172

Made in the USA
Lexington, KY
10 September 2015